GROWING UP IN A LESBIAN FAMILY

DATE DUE

GROWING UP IN A LESBIAN FAMILY

Effects on Child Development

Fiona L. Tasker
Susan Golombok

THE GUILFORD PRESS
New York   London

©1997 The Guilford Press
A Division of Guilford Publications, Inc.
72 Spring Street, New York, NY 10012

Printed in the United States of America

This book is printed on acid-free paper.

Last digit is print number: 9   8   7   6   5   4   3   2

Library of Congress Cataloging-in-Publication Data
Tasker, Fiona L.
  Growing up in a lesbian family : effects on child development /
Fiona L. Tasker, Susan Golombok.
      p.   cm.
    Includes bibliographical references and index.
    ISBN 1-57230-170-8 (hard)—ISBN 1-57230-412-X (pbk.)
    1. Children of gay parents—United States.   2. Lesbian mothers—
United States—Family relationships.   3. Child development—United
States.   4. Gender identity—United States.   5. Sex role—United
States.   I. Golombok, Susan.   II. Title.
HQ777.8.T39   1997
306.874'3—DC21   96-444471
                                                                          CIP

To our mothers

Acknowledgments

The longitudinal study we discuss in this book began in the mid-1970s, and there are many people who have been influential in its development along the way. Our grateful thanks to all those who have contributed, including those we have no space to mention individually. In particular, a special acknowledgment should be given to the families who enthusiastically participated in the original research project and in the subsequent follow-up study. The insights of both parents and children have motivated us to write this book and increased our understanding of this topic.

We were also fortunate to have much practical help with the research. The project was generously funded by the Wellcome Trust (U.K.). For the follow-up study, the staff of the Office of Population Censuses and Surveys, the National Health Central Register, many family health services authorities, and many individual general practitioners all helped us in tracing families with whom we had lost contact over the years.

There are many colleagues and friends at City University, London and elsewhere who have shared with us their ideas and given their unstinting support to the project. We are grateful to Michael Rutter for his advice and encouragement in the original and follow-up studies. Anne Spencer deserves a special mention for her contribution to the initial research. John Rust generously gave us the benefits of his statistical wisdom. Andy MacLeod provided thoughtful encouragement during the follow-up study. We are also grateful to Charlotte Patterson for her perceptive comments on the manuscript. Finally, we would like to thank Clare Murray for her thoughts on the research and help with coding the data, and Margaret Pain for her invaluable administrative skills.

Contents

GROWING UP IN A LESBIAN FAMILY

CHAPTER ONE

Introduction

IN THIS book we describe our study of the experiences of children raised by lesbian mothers. When we first began the study, in 1976, the children were around 10 years old. We interviewed them again in 1991, at the age of around 25 years. This is the first study to have followed the sons and daughters of lesbian mothers from childhood into adulthood and to examine the impact of their childhood experiences upon their adult lives. There has been much speculation about the consequences for children of being raised by a lesbian mother, speculation that is often based on little more than stereotypes of lesbian mothers, which, like all stereotypes, bear little resemblance to reality, and on false assumptions about the psychological processes involved in child development. We attempt to provide some insight into life in a lesbian-headed home from the perspective of those who grew up in one. These young people told us about themselves as adults and reflected upon their childhood and adolescent years.

It is not known how many lesbian mothers there are. Many lesbian women are not open about their sexual orientation for fear of rejection by family and friends and discrimination at work and in their community. Lesbian women who are mothers have the additional concern that they may lose their children in custody disputes or that their children may be taken into foster care. Nevertheless, estimates have been made of the number of lesbian mothers in the United States, and these range from 1 to 5 million (Falk, 1989; Patterson, 1992). The majority became mothers in the context of a heterosexual marriage. Some lesbians are aware of their attraction toward women from adolescence whereas others are unaware of their feelings toward women until they become involved in a lesbian relationship, a relationship that commonly evolves from a close friendship. Some lesbian mothers remain married, either refraining from acting upon their feelings toward women or having lesbian relationships while continuing to live with their husband. Others divorce, either to live alone or to live with a female partner. When the mother establishes a home with her partner, the children gain a stepparent — and sometimes stepsiblings as well.

Lesbian mothers first became a focus of public attention in the 1970s following a rise in the number of child custody disputes involving a lesbian mother; these were women who had given birth to their children within the early years of marriage, and before coming out as lesbian.

In custody disputes between heterosexual parents, it is generally the mother who is awarded care and control of her children. When the mother is lesbian, however, custody is commonly denied. Whereas the likelihood of a lesbian mother retaining custody may be slightly higher in the 1990s than it was in the 1970s (Rivera, 1991), it remains the case that many lesbian mothers who go to court are unsuccessful in their quest to keep their children. For this reason, many women do not even try (Brophy, 1992).

The decision of which parent to award custody to is generally based upon which option is considered to be in the best interests of the child. But how does the judge decide which is best? When a custody dispute involves a lesbian mother, her sexual orientation often becomes the major focus of the case at the expense of factors that are usually taken into account, namely, the continuity and quality of the mother–child relationship. It is generally assumed that if children remain with their lesbian mother, negative consequences will ensue. All kinds of assumptions have been made in courtrooms about the difficulties children are likely to experience as a result of being raised by a lesbian mother, and little attention has been paid to what is actually known about such children (Kleber, Howell, & Tibbits-Kleber, 1986; Falk, 1989; Editors of the Harvard Law Review, 1990; Green, 1992). We shall take a look at these assumptions and examine their validity in the light of findings from empirical studies of families with lesbian mothers.

RESEARCH ON LESBIAN-LED FAMILIES

First, a word about the research. Most studies of lesbian-led families have compared children in these households with children in households headed by a single heterosexual mother (e.g., Hoeffer, 1981; Kirkpatrick, Smith, & Roy, 1981; Golombok, Spencer, & Rutter, 1983; Green, Mandel, Hotvedt, Gray, & Smith, 1986; Huggins, 1989). These two types of family are alike in that the children are being raised by women without the presence of a father, but they differ in the sexual orientation of the mother. Since most of the children in these studies were born into a heterosexual marriage, the children in the two types of family also share the experience of parental separation or divorce. Thus, any differences that exist between children in these lesbian and heterosexual mother families may be attributed to the mother's sexual orientation. This research has examined the areas of child development that have been the focus of concern in custody cases: gender development, emotional development, and social development. In the following paragraphs we present the broad conclusions from this body of research. A more detailed discussion is available in reviews by Falk (1989), Tasker and Golombok (1991), Golombok and Tasker (1994), and Patterson (1992, 1995a).

Children's Gender Development

In examining the processes involved in gender development, a distinction is generally made between gender identity, gender role, and sexual orientation. *Gender identity* is one's concept of oneself as male or female, as reflected in the statements "I am a boy" or "I am a girl." *Gender role* includes the behaviors and attitudes that are considered to be appropriate for males and females in a particular culture. In the western world, girls who enjoy dolls and playing house and boys who enjoy rough sports, fighting, and playing with cars, trucks, and guns are considered to show typical sex role behavior. However, there is a great deal of overlap between the preferred activities and interests of boys and girls, and there is much variation within each group as well. *Sexual orientation* refers to a person's sexual attraction, which may be toward those of the opposite sex (heterosexual sexual orientation), the same sex (lesbian or gay male sexual orientation), or both (people who are sexually attracted to both women and men are bisexual).

Gender identity, gender role, and sexual orientation relate to each other in different ways. Gender identity is almost always in line with the person's biological sex; biological males develop a male gender identity and biological females develop a female gender identity. For a very small minority of people, known as transsexuals, the two do not match. When this happens, a person who is physically male feels that "he" is really a "she"; it is even less common for a person with a female body to have a male gender identity, that is , to feel that "she" is really a "he." Male-to-female transsexuals (who are physically male) often describe themselves as "a woman trapped in a man's body," and female-to-male transsexuals (who are physically female) feel that they are men trapped in a women's body. The sexual orientation of transsexual men and women may be heterosexual, homosexual, or bisexual.

For the vast majority of people whose gender identity is consistent with their biological sex, gender identity is linked to gender role, although the extent of the association between the two varies from one person to another. Some girls with a female gender identity may show feminine gender role behavior in terms of the way they dress and the activities they prefer; others may have interests that are more commonly associated with boys but feel quite sure that they are girls. Just because children do not adhere to prescribed gender roles does not mean that they are uncertain about their gender identity. However, there is a very small minority of children who are classified by the American Psychiatric Association (1994) as having "gender identity disorder of childhood"; these children express a strong desire to be the opposite sex and characteristically engage in cross-gender behavior.

Knowing a person's sexual orientation does not tell you about his or her gender role. Lesbian women may show traditionally feminine or traditionally masculine gender role behavior, just as heterosexual women do, and the same is true of gay and heterosexual men. Whatever people's sexual orientation, their gender identity remains in line with their biological sex (unless they are transsexual). Lesbian women, like heterosexual women, have no doubt that they are female, and gay men, like heterosexual men, have no doubt that they are male. The gender identity of most bisexual men and women also matches their biological sex.

What does existing research tell us about the gender identity, gender role behavior, and sexual orientation of children raised by lesbian mothers? First, the gender identity of such children is in line with their biological sex. In none of the children studied to date, estimated by Patterson (1992) to be more than 300, has there been evidence of gender identity disorder; all of the boys are sure that they are male, and all of the girls are sure that they are female. None of the children wishes to be the other sex or consistently engages in cross-gender behavior.

In terms of gender role, no differences have been found between children in the two types of family for either boys or girls. In fact, examination of preferred toys, games, activities, and friendships shows the children in both types of family to be quite traditional. In one study (Hoeffer, 1981), a careful investigation was made of the relationship between the children's toy and activity preferences and those preferred by their mother. Interestingly, it was found that the mothers' preferences had little impact on the preferences of their children. Lesbian mothers' greater preference, compared to heterosexual mothers, for an equal mixture of masculine and feminine toys for their children had little influence on the toys and activities chosen by their daughters and sons.

One of the most commonly voiced assumptions in child custody cases involving a lesbian mother is that the children will grow up to be homosexual, an outcome that is generally considered to be undesirable by those involved in decision making in courts of law. Until the present time, studies of lesbian-led families have focused on children rather than adults; as a result there has been little research evidence either to support or to refute this claim. One exception is Gottman's (1990) study of adult daughters of lesbian and heterosexual mothers. In that study approximately 16% of the young women identified themselves as lesbian; the proportion of daughters who identified themselves as lesbian was similar for the two types of family. Adult sons of gay fathers were investigated by Bailey, Bobrow, Wolfe, and Mikach (1995), who found that more than 90% were heterosexual. In a study of adolescent children of lesbian and heterosexual mothers, only one child of a heterosexual mother identified as homosexual (Huggins, 1989). Our current study of adults raised as children by lesbian mothers has the advantage of providing an opportunity to explore this issue in a sample of young adults who were recruited to the study *before* their sexual orientation was established. Findings relating to the sexual orientation of these young people are presented in Chapter 6.

Children's Emotional Development

Two studies have examined the assumption that children raised in lesbian households experience emotional or behavioral difficulties as a result of their upbringing, and neither has produced any evidence that this assumption is valid. The presence of psychiatric difficulties in the child was assessed by means of an interview with the mother in a study by Golombok et al. (1983) which compared children from lesbian-led families with children brought up by a single heterosexual mother. The interview had been specifically designed for this purpose, and its ability to reliably detect the most commonly occurring childhood disorders had been demonstrated in previous research (Graham & Rutter, 1968; Cox & Rutter, 1985). For each child a rating was made of whether or not there was evidence of psychiatric disorder; where disorder was present, a diagnosis of the type of disorder (e.g., emotional disorder or conduct disorder) was given. These ratings were made by a child psychiatrist who was not told whether the child was from a family with a lesbian or a single heterosexual mother. Examination of the findings showed that there were no differences in psychiatric state between the children of lesbian and heterosexual mothers. If anything, there was a trend toward more difficulties among the children reared by a heterosexual mother: eight children (out of a total of 38) in single heterosexual mother families had a definite psychiatric problem compared with two (out of a total of 37) in lesbian mother families, and it was found that five children in the single heterosexual mother group had been referred for psychiatric treatment as compared with only one in the lesbian mother group. In addition to interviewing the mothers, the researchers asked schoolteachers to complete a questionnaire measure of the children's emotional and behavioral problems. Again, there was no difference in the incidence of difficulties between the two groups of children; the sons and daughters of lesbian mothers were no more likely to show emotional or behavioral problems than were children in single heterosexual mother families. Since mothers may have wished to conceal their children's problems, the information obtained from schoolteachers provides important validation of the mothers' reports.

Similar findings regarding children's emotional well-being were reported by Kirkpatrick et al. (1981). Ratings of psychiatric disorder, based upon information obtained during an interview with the mother, were made by a child psychiatrist who was unaware of the family background of the child. There was no difference between groups in the proportion of children rated as showing a disorder, with approximately 10% of children in both families headed by lesbian mothers and those headed by single heterosexual mothers receiving a psychiatric diagnosis.

An important aspect of human development, one that is closely related to psychological well-being, is the development of self-esteem. No differences in levels of self-esteem have been demonstrated between the offspring of lesbian and single heterosexual mothers, either in childhood (Puryear, 1983) or in adolescence (Huggins, 1989). It seems, therefore, from research on emotional well-being during childhood and on self-esteem during childhood and adolescence that children in lesbian mother families are at no greater risk for emotional or behavioral problems than children raised by their mother in comparable heterosexual households. Thus, the concerns raised in law courts that children raised by lesbian mothers will experience psychological difficulties are not supported by existing empirical evidence. Nevertheless, it has sometimes been suggested that their difficulties will emerge when they reach adulthood. This issue is addressed in Chapter 7.

Children's Social Development

An objection to granting lesbian mothers custody of their children stems from the concern, which is invariably raised during custody proceedings, that the children will be teased about their mother's sexual orientation and ostracized by their peers. The fear is that this situation will be deeply upsetting to children and will have a negative effect on their ability to form and maintain friendships. The mothers in the study by Golombok et al. (1983) were interviewed to obtain systematic information on the quality of their children's friendships and interactions with peers. These ratings were made by a rater who was not informed of the child's family background. No differences in the quality of their friendships were identified between children raised by lesbian and by single heterosexual mothers. Only two children in each group showed definite difficulties involving personal distress, social impairment, or restricted activities, and a further one-third in each group showed minor difficulties associated with shyness, difficulty in maintaining friendships, or quarreling. In the investigation by Green et al. (1986) no group differences were found for children's perceptions of their popularity with peers or for mothers' ratings of their children's sociability and social acceptance. It seems either that stigmatization by peers is not a major problem for children of lesbian mothers or at least that exposure to teasing or ostracism does not prevent them from forming meaningful and rewarding friendships.

Children may be teased about a wide range of characteristics relating either to themselves or to their families. Children are teased about their size, their shape, their religion, their race—generally about whatever makes them different from the accepted norm. It seems likely, therefore, that many boys and girls in families led by lesbian mothers will at some time be subjected to distressing comments, and even to bullying, about their mother's lesbian identity. While existing studies show that children of lesbian mothers are generally accepted by their peers and form close friendships, the majority of the children in these studies had not yet reached adolescence. In Chapter 5 we report on young adults' recollections of, and responses to, stigmatization in their teenage years.

LESBIAN MOTHERS AND THE COURTS

In courts of law, lesbian mothers have been deemed unsuitable as parents on a number of grounds (see Arnup, 1995, for a critical review of U.S. and Canadian legislation affecting lesbian mothers). It has been argued that they are emotionally unstable and prone to psychiatric disorder, that they are not maternal, and that they, or their partner, might sexually abuse their children. In fact, there is no evidence to support any of these claims. It is well established that lesbian women, whether or not they are mothers, are at no greater risk for psychiatric disorder than heterosexual women (e.g., Bell & Weinberg, 1978). It has also been demonstrated that lesbian mothers are just as child oriented (Miller, Jacobsen, & Bigner, 1981), just as warm and responsive to their children (Golombok et al., 1983), and just as nurturant and confident (Mucklow & Phelan, 1979) as their heterosexual counterparts. And, contrary to the view expressed in a number of custody cases that the relationship with the lesbian mother's female partner will take priority over child care, the day-to-day life of lesbian mothers is just as centered around their children as is that of heterosexual mothers (Pagelow, 1980; Kirkpatrick et al., 1981). After divorce, lesbian mothers are more concerned than heterosexual mothers that their children should have contact with men (Kirkpatrick et al., 1981), and children raised by lesbian mothers following divorce see their fathers more frequently than do children raised by divorced heterosexual mothers (Golombok et al., 1983). While there are no empirical studies of the sexual abuse of children by lesbian mothers, Patterson (1992) reminds us that in the large majority of cases of sexual abuse the perpetrators are male (Finkelhor & Russell, 1984).

Recent research has focused less on establishing whether or not lesbian mothers and their children differ from heterosexual mothers and their children and has instead examined which aspects of family life are most beneficial to the child and which are most detrimental. Some children live alone with their lesbian mother whereas others live with their mother and her partner. Although the assumption of the courts has generally been that the former situation is preferable, experts who have addressed this question have concluded that the opposite is more likely to be true (Golombok et al., 1983; Kirkpatrick, 1987; Huggins, 1989). As yet this issue has not been studied directly, and the experts' conclusions are based more on their impressions than on clear-cut empirical findings. It has also been suggested by both clinicians and researchers that the earlier mothers discuss their lesbian identity with their sons and daughters, the better it is for the children. Children who learn of their mother's sexual orientation before they reach adolescence seem to find it easier to deal with the issues that arise than do those who are told during their teenage years (Paul, 1986; Pennington, 1987; Patterson, 1992). In our follow-up study, the men and women we interviewed talked about their reactions to learning about their mother's sexual orientation and, where relevant, their relationship with their mother's partner. These findings are reported in Chapter 4.

In spite of the many assumptions concerning children's emotional, social, and gender development, which have resulted in lesbian mothers' losing custody of their children, no causal connection has been established between a mother's lesbian sexual orientation and negative consequences for her child. Often, children have been removed from a mother who has been responsible for their day-to-day care from birth to reside with a father with whom they have had little previous involvement. This outcome is particularly likely when the father has a new female partner and thus offers a traditional family environment (Brophy, 1989). As Hitchins and Kirkpatrick (1986) point out, it is removing a child from the home of the primary psychological parent, not the sexual orientation of that parent, that is likely to cause harm to the child.

The decision to deny a lesbian mother custody of her children has often been made in the absence of expert evidence. When experts have been called, the witness produced on behalf of the father has generally proposed, on the basis of psychoanalytic theory, that if the children remain with their mother, they are likely to experience psychological difficulties. In contrast, the expert produced on behalf of the mother has usually argued, on the basis of empirical research, that this is unlikely to be so. In the face of these opposing opinions, the judge commonly opts for the family environment that most closely approaches the traditional nuclear family and ignores the fact that one expert's view is founded on systematic research on what actually happens to children in families headed by a lesbian mother whereas the other expert is simply speculating from one particular theoretical viewpoint. As we shall see in the next chapter, different psychological theories place different degrees of emphasis on the role of parents in child development and not all predict negative developmental outcomes for children of lesbian mothers.

PLANNED FAMILIES
LED BY LESBIAN MOTHERS

In recent years a growing number of lesbian women have become parents after coming out. While some embark upon motherhood alone, many couples plan a family together and share the parenting role (Patterson, 1992). Pregnancy is sometimes achieved through heterosexual intercourse, but often donor insemination is chosen as the means of conception. The donor may be a friend, a relative, or an acquaintance of the biological mother or her partner and may or may not remain in contact with the family as the child grows up. Other women prefer to use semen from an anonymous donor. Self-insemination is a straightforward procedure that can be performed without the assistance of the medical profession (A. Martin, 1993; Saffron, 1994). However, a difficulty with this option is that since the anonymous donor cannot be medically screened, a current or an inherited illness may inadvertently be passed on to the child. For this reason, some women decide to have donor insemination at a clinic. The problem here is that many clinics refuse to accept women without a male partner.

Another way in which a woman who is lesbian may become a mother is through adoption (Ricketts & Achtenberg, 1990). Since in most countries and in most U.S. states lesbian couples are not permitted to adopt a child together in the way that heterosexual couples can, only one lesbian partner may become the legal parent. In the United States only if the couple lives in California or New York is joint adoption allowed. In some places it is illegal even for a single lesbian woman to adopt a child. Moreover, legislation that permits lesbian women to adopt does not guarantee that this will be an easy process: In the states of California and New York, where it is illegal to reject a prospective adoptive parent on the grounds of sexual orientation, social workers who are opposed to lesbian women becoming adoptive parents may find other ostensible reasons for not placing a child in a lesbian household (A. Martin, 1993).

Those who are against lesbian women becoming adoptive mothers raise the same objections as those who wish to prevent lesbian mothers from being granted custody of their biological children. In addition, it is argued that since children who have been put up for adoption are particularly vulnerable to emotional and behavioral problems, they should be placed in as traditional a family environment as possible. As A. Martin (1993) points out, it is ironic that when lesbian women are permitted to become adoptive parents, it is generally children who need the most skilled parenting who are placed in their care.

When lesbian partners wish to raise a family together as coparents, a decision has to be made about which partner will give birth to or will legally adopt the child. Sometimes both partners decide to have a child. However much the couple may wish to share the upbringing of a child, in most lesbian-headed homes only one woman may be the legal parent. For this reason, a common problem facing lesbian co-parents is that the nonbiological or the nonadoptive mother is not viewed by society as being a real parent (Green, 1987). This situation presents a particular difficulty if the legal mother dies or becomes incapacitated or if the partners separate and cannot agree on custody and visitation/access issues. In these circumstances the co-parent, who may have been actively involved in mothering from the moment of birth or from the time of adoption, has no legal claim over the child. This has been highlighted in recent child custody cases in which the co-parent has been denied custody or visitation/access rights or these rights have been achieved only after difficult and acrimonious litigation (Polikoff, 1990). As Polikoff points out, removing children whose biological mother has died from their sole surviving parent can cause extreme distress, as can the severance of bonds between children and their nonbiological mother when the partners break up. She argues that in order to protect the best interests of the child, courts should move away from the traditional but narrow definitions of family and parenthood and toward a definition that recognizes functional parenting (i.e., nonbiological parenting relationships that involve caregiving and responsibility for the child). Polikoff believes that parenthood should be redefined to include "anyone in a functional parental relationship that a legally recognized parent created with the intent that an additional parent–child relationship exist." Another solution to the problem of the nonbiological lesbian mother's lack of parental status is for her to adopt the child, thus making both partners legal parents (A. Martin, 1993). However, this option is not currently available to the majority of lesbian mothers.

COMPARING CHILDREN OF LESBIAN AND HETEROSEXUAL COUPLES

Although most research on lesbian-led families has focused on children who were born before their mother identified herself as lesbian, studies of children born to and raised by women who previously identified themselves as lesbian are now beginning to appear. In an investigation of preschool children, no differences between children born to lesbian couples by donor insemination and those born to heterosexual couples were found for the presence of emotional problems or difficulties in separation from the mother (Steckel, 1987). However, when the children in families headed by single heterosexual mothers were compared to the children of lesbian mothers, the former were found to be more aggressive and the latter more affectionate and responsive. In an uncontrolled clinical study by McCandlish (1987), preschool children of lesbian mothers were reported to form secure attachments to both mothers and showed no evidence of psychological difficulties.

Children between the ages of 4 and 9 years who had been born to or adopted by lesbian mothers were not found to differ from children of heterosexual parents on measures of social competence, behavior problems, sex role behavior, or the extent to which they saw themselves as aggressive, sociable, or likely to enjoy being the center of attention (Patterson, 1994). Two differences between the children of lesbian and heterosexual parents were shown: Children in lesbian mother families reported more negative reactions to stress (such as anger and fear) and a greater sense of well-being (joy and contentment) than did children in heterosexual mother families. Patterson suggests that these differences may result either from greater stress in their everyday lives or from their greater ability to acknowledge both positive and negative aspects of their emotional experience. Interestingly, of the 26 children brought up by lesbian couples, the most well-adjusted children were those from lesbian families in which both women shared responsibility for child care (Patterson, 1995b).

No differences in either cognitive functioning or behavioral adjustment were identified between children who had been conceived by donor insemination and raised by lesbian couples and a control group of children from heterosexual two-parent families (Flaks, Ficher, Masterpasqua, & Joseph, 1995). Similarly, an investigation in the United Kingdom of children raised in lesbian two-parent and single parent families from infancy showed that the mothers' lesbian sexual orientation did not have a negative impact upon either their quality of parenting or their children's psychological well-being (Golombok, Tasker, & Murray, in press). In fact, compared with mothers in two-parent heterosexual families, lesbian mothers who lived with their partner showed greater warmth and greater interaction with their children and less frequent disputes with daughters, and their children showed greater security of attachment as assessed by the Separation Anxiety Test (Klagsbrun & Bowlby, 1976).

As yet, there have been too few studies of the children of women who came out as lesbian before becoming mothers to give a clear picture of the similarities and differences between these families and other family types. It is very likely, however, that the findings of research on these families in the years to come will challenge our most deep-seated assumptions about the ways in which parents influence their children's social, emotional, and gender development.

CHAPTER TWO

Parental Influences
on Child Development

THIS CHAPTER examines what is known about the influence of heterosexual mothers on the social, emotional, and sexual identity development of their children, enabling us to view the findings of the present study of young adults raised by lesbian mothers in the wider context of current knowledge about parents and their children. As discussed in the previous chapter, it has been argued that children who grow up in a family led by a lesbian mother will be disadvantaged in terms of their social and emotional well-being and will also differ with respect to adult sexual orientation from children raised by a heterosexual mother. Whether or not this may be the case depends upon the extent to which parents are influential in these specific aspects of their children's development.

PARENTAL INFLUENCES ON CHILDREN'S
SOCIOEMOTIONAL DEVELOPMENT

What aspects of the mother–child relationship are most conducive to the child's optimum social and emotional development? Do lesbian mothers differ from heterosexual mothers in these respects? While the experiences of children with lesbian mothers will be somewhat different from those of children with heterosexual mothers, it is important to establish whether the two family types differ in ways that are likely to have implications for the social and emotional well-being of the sons and daughters who grow up in them.

The most comprehensive account of the role of the mother–child relationship in children's social and emotional development comes from attachment theory, put forward by Bowlby (1969, 1973, 1980) and Ainsworth (1972, 1982; Ainsworth, Blehar, Waters, & Wall, 1978). According to this view, the course of a child's social and emotional development is closely related to the type of attachment (i.e., secure or insecure) he or she develops to the mother during infancy, with more positive psychological outcomes generally resulting for those who experience a secure attachment relationship. It seems that securely attached children do better in a variety of ways: They are more sociable and more popular with their peers, are more sociable with strange adults, have higher self-esteem, are less aggressive, show fewer behavioral problems, and are more empathic toward others (Matas, Arend, & Sroufe, 1978; Londerville & Main, 1981; Pastor, 1981; Slade, 1987; Sroufe, Fox, & Pancake, 1983; Lewis, Feiring, McGuffog, & Jaskir, 1984; Lutkenhaus, Grossmann, & Grossmann, 1985; Suess, Grossmann, & Sroufe, 1992; Youngblade & Belsky, 1992).

The main determinant of whether the child develops a secure attachment relationship with the mother is believed to be the quality of interaction between the mother and the child. Ainsworth (1979) described mothers of securely attached infants as sensitive to the infant's signals, responsive to the infant, and emotionally expressive (i.e., often smiling, using her voice expressively and frequently touching the infant). Recent research provides empirical evidence in support of this view (Grossmann, Grossmann, Spangler, Suess, & Unzer, 1985; Smith & Pederson, 1988; Pederson et al., 1990; Isabella & Belsky, 1991; Izard, Haynes, Chisholm, & Baak, 1991). For example, it has been demonstrated that secure attachment relationships are fostered by mothers who are responsive to their infant's vocalizations and distress signals (Isabella, Belsky, & von Eye, 1989).

While studies of attachment have traditionally focused on the development of attachment in infancy, in recent years attention has turned to the examination of attachment relationships in the later years. As a result, interest in the representational aspects of attachment has grown. Through their early experiences, children are believed to form internal representations (internal working models) of their attachment relationships with their parents (Bowlby, 1969, 1973, 1980). The child's internal working model of an attachment figure, for example, as available and responsive in the case of securely attached children or as unavailable and unresponsive in the case of insecurely attached children, is believed to influence not only the child's expectations of and behavior toward that person but also his or her internal representation of the self. Thus, a child who perceives attachment figures as responsive and emotionally available is likely to hold an internal model of the self as lovable whereas a child with internal models of attachment figures as unresponsive and unavailable is likely to represent the self as unworthy of being loved. The child's internal representations of attachment figures and of the self are believed to have a profound influence on his or her relationships with others during childhood and in adult life. There is growing empirical evidence in support of Bowlby's concept of internal models of attachment relationships (e.g., Main, Kaplan, & Cassidy, 1985). It has also been demonstrated that a connection exists between internal models of attachment figures and internal models of the self (Cassidy, 1988).

Another aspect of parenting that influences the social and emotional well-being of the child is parenting style. There is a large body of research (Baumrind, 1971) to show that parents who are authoritative in style (parents who combine firm control with warmth and acceptance of the child) are more likely to have well-adjusted children than either authoritarian parents (parents who are very controlling and show little warmth) or permissive parents (parents who show much warmth and acceptance of the child but little discipline). Maccoby and Martin (1983) further distinguished between two types of permissive parents; those who are indulgent (showing high warmth and low control) and those who are neglectful (showing low warmth and low control). Using Maccoby and Martin's fourfold categorization, researchers studying families with adolescent children have recently presented findings similar to those from the earlier investigations of families with younger children (Lamborn, Mounts, Steinberg, & Dornbusch, 1991; Steinberg, Lamborn, Darling,

Mounts, & Dornbusch, 1994). In comparison with their counterparts from authoritarian, indulgent, or neglectful families, adolescents from authoritative homes showed the highest levels of psychosocial adjustment and the lowest levels of emotional distress and problem behavior. Neglectful parenting was associated with the most negative outcomes for children.

So what does this tell us about the likely outcomes for children raised in lesbian mother families? The close association between children's social and emotional development and the quality of the mother–child relationship suggests that children in lesbian mother families do not experience difficulties provided they have a positive relationship with their mother. It is important to remember, however, that the mother–child relationship does not take place within a social vacuum. External environmental factors, such as the mother's access to social support, have been shown to influence the formation of secure attachment relationships in heterosexual mother families (Crockenberg, 1981). It is conceivable that the specific pressures to which lesbian mothers are exposed, such as possible disapproval from family members, and prejudice on the part of members of the local community, may interfere with effective parenting, particularly for lesbian mothers who are not part of a supportive social network.

Growing attention has been paid in recent years to the social context of families and to the processes through which hostile social environments may disrupt family relationships. In considering the consequences for children of growing up in a lesbian mother family, one should not ignore the potential effects of an inhospitable social environment in terms not only of how it may impact upon the mother–child relationship but also of how it may directly affect the child. While children may have a good relationship with their lesbian mother, they may well encounter negative attitudes toward lesbian women in their wider social world. As discussed in Chapter 1, the expectation by some that children raised in a lesbian mother family will have social and emotional difficulties arises in part from the assumption that they will be teased about their mother's sexual orientation and ostracized by their peers. The concern is that this situation would be deeply upsetting to children and that it would have a negative effect on their ability to form and maintain friendships. There is wide agreement among psychologists that satisfactory relationships with peers are important for positive social and emotional development (Kupersmidt, Coie, & Dodge, 1990; Dunn & McGuire, 1992).

Because of the potential impact of the external social environment on the social and emotional development of children and young adults, it is important to separate the effects of factors that are directly related to lesbian motherhood from the effects of factors that are commonly associated with, but not unique to this particular family form. A large proportion of children who grow up in a lesbian mother family live with their mother and father during their early years and then experience parental separation or divorce. Following the separation of their biological parents, some children are raised by their mother alone, some live in a stepfamily with their mother and her female partner, and others move in and out of these two family types. Thus, apart from the acquisition of a female rather than a male stepparent for those whose mothers enter into a new cohabiting relationship, the experiences of children in lesbian mother families are in many ways similar to those likely to be encountered by any child whose parents separate or divorce. It is important to distinguish between outcomes for children that may result from circumstances that are associated with a nontraditional family environment and those that are a consequence of living in a lesbian mother family per se. That is, the social and emotional well-being of young adults in lesbian mother families should be placed in the context of their past experience of parental separation or divorce and their being subsequently reared in a nontraditional family.

Single Parenthood

Almost one-fourth of American families (Burns, 1992) and one-fifth of British families (Roll, 1992) are headed by single parents, around 90% of whom are mothers. In the large majority of one-parent families that have been studied, it is indeed the father who is most often the absent parent. Much of the early research on one-parent families suggested poor outcomes for children's cognitive, social, or emotional development. However, the methods used were often inadequate and the findings of the more carefully conducted studies tended to be inconsistent (Herzog & Sudia, 1973; Biller, 1974). A major problem was the failure to consider factors that may be associated with single parenthood but not caused by it. This is highlighted in a study of a nationally representative sample of families in the United Kingdom in which children in one- and two-parent families were compared (Ferri, 1976). Children in one-parent families were found to be less well adjusted than those with two parents. But the children raised by a single parent also experienced a number of disadvantages, such as lower socioeconomic status, poor housing, and economic hardship. When these factors were taken into account, there was little difference in emotional adjustment between the two groups of children. That is, the absence of a parent in itself was not adversely related to the child's social adjustment. Instead, it was the poverty and social isolation that accompanied single parenthood that had a negative effect. Similarly, after controlling for social class, researchers conducting large studies in the United States found no impairment in IQ in children whose fathers were absent (Broman, Nichols, & Kennedy, 1975; Svanum, Bringle, & McLaughlin, 1982).

Another problem has been the failure to take account of the reason for becoming a one-parent family. In a study comparing children whose parents had divorced or separated and those who had lost a parent through death, Rutter (1971) found a higher incidence of behavioral problems among the children who had experienced divorce or separation; he concluded that discordant family relationships, rather than the loss of a parent, were responsible for the children's difficulties. Further evidence for the importance of factors that predate the transition from a two-parent to a one-parent family comes from longitudinal studies in the United States and the United Kingdom comparing the behavior problems of children whose parents divorced or separated between the first and second clinical assessment of the child and the behavior problems of children whose families remained intact during this interval (Cherlin et al., 1991; Elliott & Richards, 1991). It was found that behavior problems and family difficulties that were present *before* the parents' separation or divorce were strongly associated with the children's difficulties after the families had broken up. Thus, it is not only what happens to children after their parents separate but also their circumstances beforehand that influence the impact of becoming a one-parent family on their emotional and social development.

It has often been argued that the lack of a father as an identification figure or role model will result in atypical sex role behavior in children, particularly for boys. For this reason, much of the research on single-parent families has focused children's sex-typed behavior. The empirical findings relating to this issue are contradictory and inconclusive (Herzog & Sudia, 1973; Biller, 1974; Stevenson & Black, 1988). Most children raised by a single mother show typical sex role development, but there may be a slight effect on some behaviors and attitudes. Boys of preschool age whose fathers are absent tend to show less stereotyped choices of toys and activities. The behavior of older father-absent boys appears to be more stereotyped than that of their father-present age-mates. This effect is strongest for aggressive behavior, which is more common among boys who have experienced parental divorce.

Divorce

The most noteworthy study of the effects on children of parental divorce is the longitudinal investigation by Hetherington and her colleagues (Hetherington, Cox, & Cox, 1982, 1985; Hetherington, 1988, 1989). Children of divorced parents in families where the mother was awarded custody were compared with children of nondivorced parents 2 months, 1 year, 2 years, and 6 years after the divorce using a variety of observational, interview, and rating scale measures of the children's behavior at home and at school. It was found that in the first year the children from divorced families showed more behavioral problems. They were more aggressive, demanding, and lacking in self-control than their counterparts in nondivorced families. Two years after the divorce the girls had adapted to their new situation and had a positive relationship with their mother provided she had not remarried. The boys, although slightly improved, still showed problems in adjustment and difficulties in their relationship with their mother; in comparison with boys in nondivorced families, they were more antisocial, aggressive, and noncompliant both at home and at school and showed difficulties in maintaining friendships and in social adjustment. By the time of the 6-year follow-up, the mothers who had not remarried continued to have good relationships with their daughters and difficult relationships with their sons. This pattern was reflected in the children's behavior. The daughters were functioning well whereas the boys were more likely than boys in nondivorced families to be noncompliant, impulsive, and aggressive.

Wallerstein and her colleagues (Wallerstein & Kelly, 1980; Wallerstein, Corbin, & Lewis, 1988; Wallerstein & Blakeslee, 1989) have carried out a longitudinal study of the effects of divorce on children from the time of the parents' separation to 10 years later. A number of methodological problems associated with this research may have led to an overestimation of the incidence and severity of psychological disturbance in the children (Elliot, Ochiltree, Richards, Sinclair, & Tasker, 1990). The sample was obtained by offering counseling in return for participation, a procedure that, in spite of the authors attempts to exclude children with psychological disturbance, likely resulted in the selection of a group of children who were experiencing more difficulties than those in other divorcing families. Moreover, since a comparison group of nondivorced families was not included, it is not possible to conclude that the problems experienced by the children resulted directly from the divorce. At 5 years following divorce, it was reported that 37% of the children were moderately to severely depressed. At the 10-year follow-up, the problems were found to persist in the form of underachievement, worry, loneliness, anger, and difficulty in forming relationships. Boys and girls showed similar levels of psychological distress 5 years after the separation, but 10 years later girls showed greater evidence of emotional difficulties than boys.

Although it is generally believed that the effects of divorce are more severe during childhood for boys than for girls, not all of the research evidence points to this conclusion. The effects of marital dissolution on children's well-being has been examined using a large, nationally representative sample from the United States (Allison & Furstenberg, 1989). Reports were obtained from parents, teachers, and the children themselves. In line with other studies, the results show that marital dissolution has pervasive and long-lasting negative effects on behavior, psychological well-being, and academic performance. There is no evidence, however, that boys are more at risk than girls. A review of divorce studies was undertaken to resolve the issue of whether boys react more adversely to divorce than girls (Zaslow, 1988, 1989). It appears that boys do not respond more negatively under all circumstances: More negative reaction in a son is likely if he is living with a mother who does not remarry. Girls fare worse than boys in families with a stepfather or where the father has custody.

Hetherington (1988, 1989) found that when intense marital conflict continues after the divorce, it can have a more harmful effect than when it occurs in intact families. Wallerstein and Kelly (1980) also found that the children with difficulties were those whose parents remained in conflict after the divorce; they concluded that whether or not a child's problems diminish is a function of whether or not divorce improves the parental relationship. The quality of the child's relationships with the parents is also an important determinant of the child's psychological adjustment. Children who have good postdivorce relationships with their parents are less likely to suffer negative effects following the divorce (Hess & Camara, 1979; Hetherington, 1988). It seems that a good relationship between the child and both the parents can protect the child from the psychological problems that can result from the experience of parental divorce.

Of particular relevance to the present investigation are the longitudinal studies that have followed children who experienced parental divorce. Research from the British National Survey of Health and Development and the National Child Development Study (the British 1946 and 1958 birth cohort studies) shows that children of divorced parents are less likely to have a college education and more likely to be unemployed or have low occupational status in adult life than their counterparts from intact families (Maclean & Wadsworth, 1988; Kuh & Maclean, 1990; Elliott & Richards, 1991). Data from the National Child Development Study also show that children of divorced parents (particularly girls) are more likely to leave home early and cohabit or marry before age 20 and that this is especially so for those whose mothers remarry (Kiernan, 1992). Adolescents from divorced backgrounds also begin dating, have sexual intercourse, and enter into committed relationships sooner than their peers from nondivorced families (Flewelling & Bauman, 1990; Tasker, 1992). However, studies of adolescents' attitudes toward marriage after parental divorce indicate that they are generally more cautious about matrimony (Tasker & Richards, 1994). If adults from divorced backgrounds do marry, they themselves are more likely to experience marital difficulties and divorce (Pope & Mueller, 1976; Kuh & Maclean, 1990), and this is particularly so for women (Glenn & Kramer, 1987). Parental divorce also continues to contribute, albeit in a small way, to reduced psychological well-being in adulthood (Glenn & Kramer, 1985; Amato & Keith, 1991b).

Stepfamilies

The literature on stepfamilies emphasizes children's difficulties in adjusting to the presence of their parent's new partner. Data from the American National Survey of Children show that children in stepfamilies are more negative about their relationship with their stepparent (particularly the stepmother) than are children from intact families when asked about their equivalent biological parent (Furstenberg, 1987). Nevertheless, little difference between intact families and stepfamilies was found in the quality of family life and family activities as reported by both children and parents. Summarizing clinical findings as well as empirical research on stepfamilies, Pasley and Ihinger-Tallman (1987) concluded that stepmother families generally experience more problematic stepparent–child relationships than do stepfather families. This appears to be so from both stepparents' and stepchildren's reports and from measures of children's psychological adjustment. Conflictual stepmother–child relationships have also been found to be more common among daughters than sons (Clingempeel & Segal, 1986).

But not all research on stepfamilies reaches the same negative conclusion. For example, there are indications that adolescent stepdaughter–stepmother relationships improve over time, with an associated benefit to the girl's psychological adjustment (Clingempeel & Segal, 1986). Similarly, after the early stages of remarriage, boys in stepfather families have fewer problems than boys in non-remarried families (Vuchinich, Hetherington, Vuchinich, & Clingempeel, 1991). If the stepfather is supportive, boys often develop a good relationship with him. On the other hand, it was found that girls in stepfather families experience greater difficulty with family relations and adjustment than girls whose mothers do not remarry and that they continue to reject their stepfather however hard he tries to develop a good relationship.

The age of the child when the parent remarries seems to be an important predictor of outcome for the child. In a study of stepfather families, Hetherington and Clingempeel (1992) found early adolescence to be a particularly difficult time. Little improvement in either the adjustment of children or in the stepfather–stepchild relationship was shown over a 26-month period.

Thus, it can be seen that the family environment in which children find themselves after parental separation or divorce has implications for their social and emotional well-being. It is important to bear in mind that the young adults in the present study moved from a two-parent heterosexual family to either a single-parent household or a stepfamily, often followed by further transitions to other family forms.

PARENTAL INFLUENCES ON CHILDREN'S GENDER DEVELOPMENT

Although it is a commonly held view that lesbian mothers are more likely than heterosexual mothers to have lesbian daughters and gay sons, opinion varies among psychological and biological theorists regarding the extent to which it is possible for parents to influence the sexual orientation of their children. At one extreme are the biological theorists who consider that parents make little difference. At the other end of the spectrum are psychoanalytic theorists who believe that relationships with parents early in childhood are central to the development of sexual orientation in adult life. In the following paragraphs various theoretical perspectives are examined in terms of their explanations of the processes involved in the development of sexual orientation, examined particularly with respect to what they tell us about the mechanisms, if any, through which parents may play a role in that development.

Biological Theories

In the 1990s we have witnessed a resurgence of interest in genetic explanations of sexual orientation. This has resulted partly from the publication of two studies, following rather different lines of research, that have pointed to a genetic influence. The first, a study of homosexual men with twin brothers, found that 52% of monozygotic co-twins were also homosexual as compared with 22% of dizygotic co-twins (Bailey & Pillard, 1991). Lesbian women with twin sisters have also been investigated by these researchers. The findings are similar to those from the study of homosexual men (Bailey, Pillard, Neale, & Agyei, 1993): Forty-eight percent of monozygotic co-twins were reported to be lesbian, in contrast with 16% of dizygotic co-twins. While the concordance found between identical twin pairs is greater than that between nonidentical twin pairs and thus suggests a genetic link to homosexuality, this does not necessarily mean that a homosexual (or heterosexual) orientation is dependent upon a specific genetic pattern. People with similar genetic patterns have similar characteristics and, as a consequence, tend to have similar life experiences. Since monozygotic twins are alike in a variety of ways, it is not surprising that this should also be the case for sexual orientation.

The second study, which has attracted a great deal of attention from the general public as well as the scientific community, claims to have identified a genetic marker for male homosexuality. Of 40 pairs of brothers, both of whom were homosexual, 33 pairs were found to have a marker in a small region of the X chromosome (Hamer, Hu, Magnuson, Hu, & Pattatucci, 1993). This suggests that there may be a specific gene, yet to be located, that is linked to male homosexuality. It does not mean, however, that the presence of this gene, if it exists, determines a homosexual orientation; instead, it may be one of many factors that influence development in a homosexual rather than a heterosexual direction. Neither does it mean that all homosexual men possess the gene. After all, the marker was not found in 7 pairs of brothers. It remains for this research to be replicated before any conclusions can be drawn from the findings. There are also many questions that must be addressed before the function of this gene can be understood. For example, is the gene found in heterosexual men? Or in lesbian women? Even if a specific gene that predisposes a person toward homosexuality is identified it is important to bear in mind that people experience other influences throughout the life span, both biological and social, that may push or pull them toward a heterosexual or a homosexual orientation.

Our sex hormones may constitute one such biological influence. While no consistent differences in sex hormone levels have been identified between heterosexual and homosexual adults (Meyer-Bahlburg, 1984), there is some evidence to suggest that the hormonal environment to which we are exposed prenatally may play some part in the development of our sexual orientation. The consequences of variations in prenatal hormone levels for sexual orientation has been examined by studying adults who were exposed in the womb to an unusually high or an unusually low level of sex hormones, either because of an inherited disorder or owing to the administration of synthetic hormones during pregnancy to women at risk for miscarriage. Studies of women with congenital adrenal hyperplasia (CAH), a genetically transmitted disorder in which malfunctioning adrenal glands produce high levels of androgens from the prenatal period onward, have found these women to be more likely than women who do not have the disorder to consider themselves bisexual or lesbian, suggesting that raised levels of androgens prenatally may predispose toward a lesbian sexual orientation (Money, Schwartz, & Lewis, 1984; Dittman, Kappes, & Kappes, 1992). In addition, women exposed prenatally to the synthetic estrogen diethylstilbestrol (DES), an androgen derivative, have been compared with unexposed women from the same clinic and with their unexposed sisters (Ehrhardt et al., 1985; Meyer-Bahlburg et al., 1995). In comparison with both control groups, the women who had been exposed to DES reported increased bisexual or lesbian responsiveness. It is important to point out that most of the women with CAH and most of the women prenatally exposed to DES were heterosexual in spite of their atypical endocrine history. In addition, some women who were classified as lesbian or bisexual had simply reported feelings of sexual attraction toward women rather than actual involvement in sexual relationships.

On the basis of the aforementioned research, together with animal research that has demonstrated that sex hormones influence the development of sex-typed behavior as well as sex differences in the structure of the brain (Goy & McEwen, 1980), it has been proposed that prenatal sex hormones may act upon neural substrates of the human brain to facilitate development toward heterosexuality or homosexuality (Money, 1987, 1988; Hines & Green, 1990). According to this view, androgenic hormones predispose both sexes toward a preference for female sexual partners while men and women who lack a critical amount of these hormones are more likely to prefer men. However, the mechanisms involved in the link between prenatal sex hormones, sex differences in brain structure, and sexual orientation have not been established (Byne & Parsons, 1993). While an anatomical difference in the hypothalamus of homosexual and heterosexual men has recently been identified (LeVay, 1991), the reason for this difference remains unknown, as does the mechanism by which it may influence sexual orientation.

Gender Nonconformity in Childhood

A number of investigations point to a relationship between non-conventional gender role behavior in childhood and adult homosexuality. In retrospective studies, differences in childhood gender role behavior have been found between homosexual and heterosexual men, with homosexual men consistently reporting greater involvement in stereotypically female activities—such as playing with dolls, dressing in girls' clothes, and preferring girls as playmates—than their heterosexual counterparts (Saghir & Robins, 1973; Whitam, 1977; Bell, Weinberg, & Hammersmith, 1981). Comparable results have emerged from retrospective research on childhood masculinity in girls: Lesbian women have been found to differ from heterosexual women in recollecting greater tomboyish behavior, more boys and fewer girls as playmates, and a greater childhood desire to be a boy (Safer & Reiss, 1975). The validity of these retrospective studies has been questioned inasmuch as gay men and lesbian women may be more likely to identify behaviors that might have a bearing on their sexual orientation whereas heterosexual men and women may not remember, or admit to, cross-gender behavior as children. However, prospective studies of children with gender identity disorder (American Psychiatric Association, 1994)—that is, children who express a strong desire to be the other sex and characteristically engage in cross-gender behavior, including a marked preference for friends of the other sex—have produced similar findings. In a follow-up study of 55 feminine boys who had been referred to a gender identity clinic in childhood or adolescence, over 70% identified themselves as homosexual in adulthood (Zuger, 1984), and a longitudinal study of 66 feminine boys and a matched group of 55 nonfeminine boys found that 68% percent of the feminine boys developed a bisexual or homosexual orientation, compared with none in the control group (Green, 1987). The identification of a link between cross-gender behavior in childhood and homosexuality in adulthood does not mean that all or even most adults who identify themselves as homosexual were nonconventional in their gender role behavior as children. In fact, retrospective studies show that a substantial proportion of gay and lesbian adults reported no or few cross-gender behaviors in childhood, and the prospective studies examined boys who had been referred to a clinic because of marked cross-gender behavior and thus were not representative of the general population of boys who become homosexual in adulthood. So even if a lesbian or gay sexual orientation may sometimes be related to gender nonconformity in childhood, it is clear that the latter does not provide a comprehensive explanation of why some people develop a homosexual, and others a heterosexual, sexual orientation.

Investigations of parental influences on childhood gender nonconformity have failed to identify a clear and consistent association between the two, either for boys (Roberts, Green, Williams, & Goodman, 1987) or for girls (Green, Williams, & Goodman, 1982; Williams, Goodman, & Green, 1985). Furthermore, while the mechanisms that underlie the relationship between childhood gender nonconformity and adult homosexuality are not understood, there is no evidence to indicate that parents play a mediating role in this relationship. Instead, it has been suggested that male homosexuality in boys with gender identity disorder may result indirectly from the influence of low levels of prenatal androgens in reducing such male sex-typed behavior as aggression and rough-and-tumble play, a behavioral modification that causes the boys to be stigmatized by same-gender peers in childhood and thus influences them toward a homosexual orientation in adulthood (Green, 1987; Friedman, 1988; Money, 1988). This theory remains speculative. By 2 or 3 years of age children begin to segregate by gender in their play and begin to engage in different play styles, with boys being more active and aggressive than girls and girls being more nurturant and vocal than boys (Maccoby & Jacklin, 1974; Maccoby, 1988; Maccoby, 1990). There is evidence to suggest that feminine boys and masculine girls are rejected by their same-gender peers (Langlois & Downs, 1980; Asher, 1990) and that rejected children often lack the opportunity to acquire the social skills that are important for social interaction in later life (Parker & Asher, 1987; Coie & Cillessen, 1993). According to Maccoby (1990), it is through contact with same-gender peers that boys and girls acquire gender-related social skills and styles of social interaction; boys and girls who are rejected by same-gender peers would be denied this form of socialization toward distinctive male and female interactive styles. Nevertheless, a direct link between cross-gender behavior in childhood, peer group rejection, and a lesbian or gay sexual orientation in adulthood has not been empirically established.

Psychoanalytic Theory

According to traditional psychoanalytic theory, gender development is rooted in the phallic stage of psychosexual development, which occurs at about 5 years of age (Freud, 1905/1953, 1920/1955, 1933/1964; Socarides, 1978). It is in order to resolve the oedipal conflict, that is, the conflict between his sexual desire for his mother and his fear of castration by his father, that a boy is believed to shift identification from the mother to the father and take on his male characteristics. The mechanisms involved in female identification are rather different and less clearly described. The resolution of the oedipal conflict in girls is be-

lieved to be driven by penis envy and involves transferring identification from the father back to the mother and adopting a female role.

For psychoanalytic theorists, a lesbian or gay sexual orientation is often viewed as a negative outcome resulting from the
unsuccessful resolution of the oedipal conflict; it is believed that
boys who continue to identify with their mother and girls who
continue to identify with their father during the oedipal period
are more likely to identify themselves as gay or lesbian, respectively, when they grow up. The quality of children's relationships
with their parents is considered to be an important determinant
of their passage through the oedipal phase. For boys, the combination of a domineering mother and a weak father is thought
to lead to a homosexual orientation. A lesbian orientation is believed to result from a girl's hostile and fearful relationship with
her mother.

Although psychoanalytically oriented theorists believe homosexuality to arise from disturbed relationships with parents, empirical studies of the influence of parent–child relationships on
the development of a gay or lesbian identity have produced inconclusive results. In a study of psychoanalysts' reports of the
family relationships of their male homosexual patients, the fathers
of these patients were described as hostile and/or distant and the
mothers as close, intimate, and dominant (Bieber et al., 1962).
With a nonpatient sample, Evans (1969) also showed a similar
pattern of a close mother and a detached father. However, Bene
(1965a) found no evidence that homosexual men who were not
in therapy were more likely than heterosexual men to have been
overprotected by, overindulged by, or strongly attached to their
mother. In a well-controlled large-scale study by Siegelman
(1974), no differences were identified in parental childrearing style
between homosexual and heterosexual men who were low on
neuroticism. Siegelman concluded that the differences in
parent–child relationships between homosexual and heterosexual men found in earlier studies were related to differences in neuroticism rather than to homosexuality per se. Studies of the
parents of lesbian women have similarly failed to produce consistent findings, although some investigations have reported
mothers of lesbian women to be dominant and fathers to be

inferior or weak (Bene, 1965b; Kaye et al., 1967; Bell et al., 1981; Newcombe, 1985).

Social Learning and Cognitive Developmental Theories

From the perspective of classic social learning theory, which focuses on the development of childhood sex-typed behavior rather than on adult sexual orientation, the two processes that are important for children's gender development are differential reinforcement and modeling (Mischel, 1966, 1970; Bandura, 1977). There is much empirical evidence to suggest that parents of preschool children treat their sons and daughters differently, although the extent to which they are producing sex-typed behavior, rather than simply responding to preexisting differences between boys and girls, remains unknown (Maccoby & Jacklin, 1974; Lytton & Romney, 1991). However, differential reinforcement by parents seems to decline once children reach school age (Lytton & Romney, 1991; Fagot & Hagan, 1991). At this stage of a child's development friends take on a more important role: Peers consistently and strongly reinforce sex-typed toy choice and play and punish cross-gender activities (Carter, 1987).

According to classic social learning theorists, boys and girls also learn sex-typed behavior by imitating models of their own gender, particularly the same-gender parent. However, the idea that children acquire sex-typed behavior by directly imitating same-gender parents is now thought to be rather simplistic, and a modified version of social learning theory has been proposed (Perry & Bussey, 1979; Bussey & Bandura, 1984; Bandura, 1986). It seems that children learn which behaviors are considered to be appropriate for males and which for females by observing many men and women and boys and girls and by noticing which behaviors are performed frequently by females and rarely by males and vice versa. Children then use these abstractions of sex-appropriate behavior as models for their own imitative performance. Thus, children observe a wide variety of role models in their daily life and tend to imitate those whom they consider to be typical of their sex. Friends, in particular, appear to be important role models; school-age boys and girls show a strong preference for same-gender peers (Maccoby, 1988). But it is gender stereotypes, rather than specific individuals, that seem to be most influential in the acquisition of sex-typed behavior. Gender stereotypes are pervasive in our society, and children are aware of these stereotypes from as early as 2 years of age (Stern & Karraker, 1989; C. L. Martin, 1991; Signorella, Bigler, & Liben, 1993).

Although social learning theorists have focused on the acquisition of sex role behavior rather than on the development of sexual orientation, the processes of reinforcement and modeling would also apply to sexual orientation to the extent that it results from social learning. Thus, heterosexual parents may encourage their children toward a heterosexual orientation by direct reinforcement, and they may act as heterosexual role models. But, as we have seen, it is not just parents who perform these functions. Peers may also reinforce sexual partner preference and may act as sexual role models, and sexual stereotypes may provide a basis for modeling as well.

Cognitive developmental theorists, like social learning theorists, have focused on the development of childhood gender identity and sex role behavior rather than on adult sexual orientation. Nevertheless, this theoretical approach can help us to explore the role of parents in the child's development into a heterosexual, lesbian, or gay adult. Early studies examined children's developing understanding of the concept of gender (Kohlberg, 1966; Stagnor & Ruble, 1987). More recently, attention has focused on the way in which children organize knowledge about gender, that is, on children's development of gender stereotypes (Martin & Halverson, 1981; C. L. Martin, 1989, 1991). Cognitive developmental explanations of gender development emphasize that children actively construct for themselves from the gendered world around them what it means to be male or female and adopt behaviors and characteristics that they perceive as being consistent with their own gender. Once again, it is gender stereotypes, not parents, that are viewed as being the primary source of gender-related information. To the extent that cognitive processes are contributing to the adoption of a heterosexual or homosexual orientation, it would seem that young people seek out information in their social world that is in line with their emerging sexual orientation and come to value and identify with those characteristics that are consistent with their view of themselves as heterosexual or homosexual.

Social Constructionist Theories

Symbolic interactionist and social constructionist approaches to the development of sexual identity start from the premise that sexual feelings are not essential qualities that the individual is born with or that are socialized by childhood experiences. What these approaches have in common is an emphasis on the individual's active role, guided by his or her culture, in structuring reality and creating sexual meanings for particular acts (Hart, 1981; Richardson, 1981; Tiefer, 1987; Kitzinger, 1995). These theorists argue that sexual identity is constructed throughout the life span; the individual first becomes aware of cultural scenarios for socially appropriate sexual encounters and then develops internal fantasies associated with sexual arousal (intrapsychic scripts) and interpersonal scripts for orchestrating specific sexual acts (Simon & Gagnon, 1987; Gagnon, 1990). It has been proposed that childhood sexual experiences such as genital play with someone of the same gender, or same-gender emotional attachments and fantasies create a potential source of information for later homosexual identification (Plummer, 1975). The possession of a particular body type and early experiences of exhibiting cross-gender behavior or of feeling different from peers are also thought to facilitate homosexual identification because of the cultural association between them and later homosexuality.

From an interactionist perspective an important part is played by identification with significant others, who enable an individual to either neutralize a homosexual potential or construct a homosexual identity. For example, parents often ignore or fail to label children's behavior as being sexual; as a result, children do not integrate these feelings into their sexual self-concept. Conversely, parents may respond negatively to what they perceive as children's sexual activity (Gagnon & Simon, 1973; Gagnon, 1977). Indeed, numerous heterosexual cultural constructions are readily available for neutralizing the meaning of same-gender erotic acts (Henecken, 1984). Plummer points out that although many people have same-gender experiences at some time in their life, few develop a homosexual identity. He proposes that for men from heterosexual families who go on to develop a homosexual identity, access to other homosexual men is important for providing a series of accounts that validates their homosexuality and for helping them develop a repertoire of appropriate behaviors for interacting with homosexual men, thus enabling them to adopt a homosexual role.

From a feminist perspective, intimate relationships are viewed not just as reflections of personal preference but as creation of and responses to patriarchal society (Cartledge & Ryan, 1983). Radical feminists argue that being a lesbian is not an essential trait but an identity that is a positive choice arising from a political rejection of heteropatriarchy (Kitzinger, Wilkinson, & Perkins, 1992; Golden, 1994; Kitzinger & Wilkinson, 1995). Different lesbian identities are viewed as resulting from different discourses in society regarding the meaning of what it is to be a lesbian from the perspective both of the lesbian herself and of prevailing ideologies (Ettore, 1980; Kitzinger, 1987). It is argued that because a heterosexual identity is assumed in our society, most young people are given no choice but to follow a heterosexual route.

CONCLUSION

So what can we conclude about the factors that influence sexual orientation? And what role, if any, is played by parents? What is clear is that no single factor has been identified as a determinant of whether people will identify themselves as heterosexual or homosexual. Instead, it seems that the pathways that lead from the prenatal period to adult sexual orientation are complex and that individuals experience a variety of biological, psychological, and cultural influences at different stages of development. As yet, there is no clear answer to the question of whether sexual orientation is biologically based. And if researchers do establish for certain that biological factors are involved, the answer is unlikely to be a simple yes. Even those who are most committed to the view that sexual orientation may be genetically or hormonally determined do not believe that biological factors operate independently of the social world in which we grow up.

Is it the case that children of lesbian mothers will be more likely than children of heterosexual mothers to be lesbian or gay? As we have seen, different predictions arise from the different theories according to the role ascribed to parents. Traditional psychoanalytic theorists, stressing the importance of the presence of heterosexual parents for the successful resolution of the oedipal conflict, would expect that the lack of a father figure, together with the mother's atypical female role, would influence the sexual orientation of a child brought up in a lesbian mother family. While studies of children raised by heterosexual parents have failed to produce empirical evidence to demonstrate that the quality of the parent–child relationships influences the development of a child's sexual orientation, a psychoanalytic theorist might predict that a gay identity would be particularly likely for boys with close relationships with their lesbian mothers and that a lesbian identity would be likely for girls with hostile relationships with their lesbian mothers. A theorist with a social learning theory perspective might postulate that the patterns of reinforcement operating in lesbian mother families differ from those in heterosexual mother families such that young people in the former are less likely to be discouraged from embarking upon lesbian or gay relationships. Although contemporary social learning theorists are less likely than classical social learning theorists to emphasize the importance of the same-gender parent as a role model, it could be argued that by virtue of their nontraditional family the sons and daughters of lesbian mothers may hold less rigid stereotypes about what constitutes acceptable male and female behavior than their peers in heterosexual mother families and thus may be more likely to consider having relationships with same-gender partners. What social learning, cognitive developmental, and social constructionist theorists have in common is the view that sexual orientation is influenced, to some extent at least, by social norms. These theorists would argue that children who grow up in an atmosphere of positive attitudes toward homosexuality can be expected to be more open to involvement in gay or lesbian relationships themselves.

CHAPTER THREE

The Longitudinal Study

THE BRITISH Longitudinal Study of Lesbian Mother Families began in the mid-1970s (Golombok et al., 1983), and the follow-up study commenced in 1990 (Tasker & Golombok, 1995; Golombok & Tasker, 1996). This chapter describes the sample of lesbian mothers and their children, the comparison group of children brought up by heterosexual mothers, methodological issues, and the techniques employed to collect and analyze data.

LESBIAN AND HETEROSEXUAL MOTHER FAMILIES IN THE INITIAL STUDY

The samples of lesbian families and heterosexual single-parent families initially participated in the study in 1976 and 1977. Similar procedures were used to recruit the two groups; advertisements in lesbian and single-parent publications and contacts with lesbian and single-parent groups. The criteria for the inclusion of lesbian mothers were that they regarded themselves as predominantly or wholly lesbian in their sexual orientation and that their current (or most recent) sexual relationship was with a woman. The heterosexual mother group was defined in terms of mothers whose most recent sexual relationship had been heterosexual but who did not have a male partner living with them at the time of the original investigation. Mothers from both groups came from different regions across the United Kingdom. Each group comprised 27 female-headed families. Of the children who participated in the study, 39 were from lesbian mother families and 39 from heterosexual mother families.[1] Out of the 27 lesbian mothers, 21 had previously been married and two had cohabited with a male partner without marriage. Of the remaining four lesbian mothers, two had become pregnant as a result of a noncohabiting relationship with a man, one had adopted her child, and the other mother, who had two children, had adopted one and conceived the other through donor insemination. None of the children obtained through donor insemination or adoption participated in the follow-up study. Of the 27 single heterosexual mothers, 21 had been previously married, two had cohabited with a male partner without marriage, and four had conceived their children as a result of noncohabiting relationships with men.

The original investigation therefore contrasted children who were being raised by lesbian mothers with a control group of children raised by single heterosexual mothers. Without a control group it would not have been possible to deduce whether children in lesbian mother families differed from their peers, since the findings could simply reflect the behavior of children in general. Furthermore, whether the difference between the group of interest and the population in general is a real one is particularly difficult to verify when only patchy data on population norms are available. At first glance, the most obvious comparison group for a study examining the well-being of children in lesbian mother families might appear to be children brought up by their mother and father in a two-parent household. However, children raised in a two-parent family who had not seen their parents separate would not have experienced the transition to a different family structure and would not have seen their mother form a relationship with a new partner. Moreover, since psychoanalytic and social cognitive theories make predictions as to the effects of father absence on children's socioemotional development, the researchers reasoned that the presence of a father in the home of the control group children would have a confounding effect on the data. For

[1]The data from two children 4 years of age and one child of 19 at the time of the original study are included at follow-up. This increased the pool of potential participants from 75 to 78. The data for these children were not previously published (Golombok et al., 1983) because the analysis was limited to school-age children only.

these reasons, the original study, like other early studies of children in lesbian mother families, included a comparison group of children living with their heterosexual single mother after their mother and father's separation (Hoeffer, 1981; Kirkpatrick et al., 1981; Green et al., 1986).

Assessments in the Original Study

In the original study, the main sources of data were provided by individual interviews with mothers and children. The researchers used adaptations of standardized interviews that had been previously developed to assess various aspects of personal and family functioning and that had been shown to have good reliability and validity (Brown & Rutter, 1966; Rutter & Brown, 1966; Rutter, Cox, Tupling, Berger, & Yule, 1975). The interviews were conducted by two female interviewers (Susan Golombok and Anne Spencer). All of the variables, together with the standardized coding scheme, are listed in Appendix I.

For both lesbian and heterosexual mother families, data were obtained from the mother's interview on the following: demographic characteristics of the family, the quality of the mother–child relationship, the mother's psychological adjustment, the child's gender role behavior, and the child's peer relationships. Standardized ratings were also made of each child's psychiatric state by a child psychiatrist who was unaware of the child's family type, according to the procedures described by Graham and Rutter (1968). In addition to the interview, each mother and her child's teacher were asked to complete the parent Rutter A Scale and teacher Rutter B Scale, respectively (Rutter et al., 1975), to assess the child's emotions, behavior and relationships. Both the A and B scales have been shown to have good reliability and to discriminate well between children with and without psychiatric disorder. Mothers also completed the Malaise Inventory, a questionnaire measure of their own mental health (Rutter, Tizard, & Whitmore, 1970). Data from both the mother's and the child's interview on the frequency with which the child engaged in a variety of sex-typed activities were used to produce a rating of the child's gender role behavior, with a high score indicating less sex-typed behavior.

A section of the interview covered issues relevant only to the lesbian mothers in the study. The main areas of interest here were the age at which the mother first became aware of her attraction to women and first had a lesbian relationship, her feelings toward men, her relationship style (monogamous or nonmonogamous), the number of years that the child had resided in a traditional heterosexual family, the child's awareness of the mother's lesbian relationships, and the mother's wishes about the child's future sexual orientation. For mothers who were cohabiting with a female partner, the division of domestic roles and child care responsibilities was examined. Ratings were also made of the quality of the couple's relationship using a standardized interview assessment of the quality of marital relationships (Quinton, Rutter, & Rowlands, 1976).

THE YOUNG ADULTS RAISED BY LESBIAN AND HETEROSEXUAL MOTHERS IN THE FOLLOW-UP STUDY

In the original study, the average age of the children was 9.5 years. Therefore, ethical considerations meant that for the follow-up study 14 years later it was necessary to first contact the mothers to request their permission to interview their children. Contact was made with 51 of the 54 mothers who had participated in the original study. During the period between the original study and follow-up, 41 of the 54 families had moved from their original address. Mothers who had moved were traced through the U.K. National Health Service Central Register and received a letter through their family doctor asking them to contact us about the study. Only three mothers and their children could not be traced in this way. In addition, one daughter had died during the intervening years. From the group of 74 potential recruits to the follow-up study, 46 young adults aged 17 to 35 were interviewed, representing a response rate of 62%. The main reasons for sample attrition appear to be the long gap between the original and follow-up studies, the sensitivity of the topic, and the change of respondent between the original study (in which mothers were the main source of data) and the follow-up study (in which the children themselves were interviewed). Eight mothers from the original lesbian mother group and eight single heterosexual mothers did not wish their family to participate in the follow-up study. This effectively excluded from the longitudinal study 11 of the children from lesbian mother families and 13 of the children from heterosexual mother families. Two of these mothers from each group said that their life had changed since the original study (details unspecified) and that they did not want their son or daughter to be reminded of an earlier time. Four of the heterosexual mothers simply returned the reply slip saying that they did not wish their family to take part. One of the lesbian mothers declined on behalf of her son, who was serving a prison sentence, and one of the heterosexual mothers declined because of family illness. Two reminder letters about the study received no reply from the remaining five lesbian mothers, and one heterosexual mother. In the end, 18 of the original group of 27 lesbian mothers and 16 of the original group of 27 single heterosexual mothers had at least one child who participated at follow-up.

When mothers consented to their family's inclusion in the follow-up study, they were reassured about the confidentiality of the information they had given in the original study. Both the lesbian and the heterosexual mothers were generally extremely helpful in encouraging their son or daughter to participate in a research interview. Young adults from both types of family were initially told that the study concerned children raised in father-absent households after their parents had separated. It was left up to the lesbian mothers to inform their children further. In all but one case, the mother was already "out" to her family. After the mothers had given their consent, only four children (one from a lesbian mother family and three from heterosexual mother families) did not participate in the research, either because they thought the interview would be too personal or because they repeatedly failed to attend appointments. One young man from a heterosexual mother family who did not wish to take part in the follow-up interview had been recently hospitalized with a diagnosis of schizophrenia.

Data from the first study were examined to ascertain the characteristics of the follow-up sample and possible reasons for sample attrition. There were no differences between follow-up participants and nonparticipants on most of the key variables from the original study: age and gender of children, mothers' social class, quality of mother–child relationship, quality of children's peer relationships, and children's gender role behavior. In addition, there were no differences between follow-up participants and nonparticipants in terms of either their own or their mother's psychological well-being at the time of or prior to the initial study. However, children who did not take part at follow-up tended to have experienced a period of separation from their mother prior to the original study (Fisher's exact test; $p = .086$). Since children were contacted through their mother, it is possible that those who had previously been separated from her may have been less likely to be in contact with her as young adults. Within the lesbian mother group, children who had been classified by their mother as probably unaware of her lesbian identity tended not to participate at follow-up ($t = -1.77$, $df = 37$, $p = .085$). Finally, children whose lesbian mother reported higher rates of interpersonal conflict with her cohabitant at the time of the original study were also less likely to contribute to the follow-up study ($t = 3.87$, $df = 19$, $p = .001$).

Twenty-five young adults from lesbian mother families (17 women and 8 men) and 21 young adults from heterosexual mother families (9 women and 12 men) took part in the follow-up study. The trend toward proportionately more young women than young men being represented in the lesbian mother group reflects the slightly higher proportion of daughters of lesbian mothers in the original study. Table 3.1 displays the demographic characteristics of the participants. The average age of the interviewees was 23.5 years with no statistically significant difference in average age between young adults from the two types of family background. No statistically significant group differences were found for either ethnicity or educational qualifications.

There were also no differences between the two groups in terms of mother's social class as assessed according to her occupation at the time of the original study. However, more of the lesbian mothers had received a college education (see Table 3.1). A number of problems are associated with the assessment of socioeconomic status for female-headed households. For example, a woman's occupational status may not be reflected in her house-

TABLE 3.1. Demographic Characteristics of Young Adults Participating in the Follow-Up Study by Family Type.

		Lesbian mother	Heterosexual single-parent mother	Fisher's exact p
Young adult's gender	Male	8	12	.078
	Female	17	9	
Young adult's ethnic group	White	23	19	NS
	Nonwhite	2	2	
Mother cohabited with new partner	Mother cohabited	22	18	NS
	No cohabitation	2	2	
Young adult's further education	Further education	14	7	NS
	No further	11	14	
Mother's socio-economic status[a]	Middle class	10	9	NS
	Working class	4	2	
Mother's further education[a]	Further education	13	5	.020
	No further education	5	11	

Note. Adapted from Golombok and Tasker (1996). Copyright 1996 by the American Psychological Association. Adapted by permission.
[a]Data are from interviews with mothers in the original study, when four of the lesbian mothers and five of the single heterosexual mothers were not in paid employment.

hold income, and her current employment may not be in line with her educational attainment (Weitzman, 1985; Maclean, 1991). Past research has linked parental educational attainment to both parenting style and parental attitudes (Hernandez, 1988; Zill, 1988), and two recent British studies of children of divorce have used maternal educational attainment as an indicator of type of parenting in the original predivorce family (Kuh & Maclean, 1990; Cockett & Tripp, 1994). Therefore, the mother's educational level (i.e., whether or not she had received higher education), rather than her occupation, was used as the measure of social class throughout the study.

By the time of the follow-up, all but one of the original control group of single heterosexual mothers were reported by their children to have had at least one heterosexual relationship and in all but two cases the mother had cohabited with or married her new male partner (see Table 3.1). Among the 25 young adults raised in lesbian mother families, 22 had lived with their mother and her female partner. Therefore, in the follow-up study the group of young adults raised by heterosexual mothers no longer functioned as a control group for father absence. Instead, they now effectively controlled for the presence of an additional parent figure in the household.

Assessments in the Follow-Up Study

Data for the follow-up study were obtained from individual interviews with the young adults raised in lesbian and heterosexual mother families. A semistructured interview schedule was developed together with a standardized coding scheme, thus keeping the same style of interview as in the original investigation. The aims of the interview were to use flexible, personally tailored questioning to collect relevant information from all respondents and to then rate all participants according to an identical coding scheme. This means that standardized data were systematically collected from both groups of young adults while the flexibility of the semistructured interview allowed respondents to recount their own experiences and feelings. Thus, we were able to increase the validity of the data collected in this previously uncharted research area.

The interview protocol covered four main areas of interest: family relationships, peer relationships, intimate relationships, and psychological adjustment. Prior to the follow-up study, the interview procedure was tested on 10 men and women from heterosexual mother families and five young people from lesbian-headed homes. Further details of the information obtained by interview are presented alongside the results in each of the following four chapters. A list of the follow-up study variables, together with their coding criteria, is given in Appendix II.

Fourteen randomly selected interviews out of the 46 conducted in the follow-up study were coded by a second interviewer in order to calculate interrater reliability. Phi coefficients and Pearson product–moment coefficients were calculated for all of the variables (listed along with each variable in Appendix II). Variables that failed to reach an interrater reliability of $r = .65$ were excluded from the statistical analyses. Although test–retest data on the long-term reliability of the interview does not exist for the present data set, comparable semistructured interviews have been shown to have acceptable long-term stability (Brown & Rutter, 1966; Rutter & Brown, 1966; Quinton et al., 1976).

The follow-up interviews took place either at the young adult's home or at the university. Participants were recompensed for any travel or other expenses they had incurred. The interviews lasted 2½ hours on average and were conducted by a female interviewer (Fiona Tasker). Each interviewee was seen alone. When arrangements for the interview were being discussed, potential participants were told that the interview covered their family history, friendships at school, health, work, and relationships. Confidentiality and the right to refuse to answer any particular questions were emphasized when discussing the appointment and again before the interview began. None of those agreeing to be interviewed refused to answer any of the questions put during the interview, although some respondents were more defensive than others.

The aim of the interview was to obtain comparable information from the young adults raised by lesbian and heterosexual mothers so that all participants could be rated on the same variables. For questions on the quality of family relationships, career history, and psychological adjustment, ensuring the equivalence of information gathered for both groups was reasonably straightforward. For other parts of the interview, however, comparability was more difficult to achieve. For example, young adults from lesbian households generally appeared to have thought about their own sexual orientation to a greater extent than did those from heterosexual mother families; consequently, they were not surprised that the interview section on close relationships included questions on this topic. In contrast, many of those from heterosexual backgrounds appeared never to have reflected on possible instances of same-gender sexual attraction prior to the interview and therefore probably did not give such considered responses. Furthermore, this problem was compounded in some cases by the interviewee's obvious embarrassment at discussing sexual feelings and the possibility of experiencing attraction toward someone of the same gender. This was true in Jim's case:

F. T.: Can you ever remember looking at pornographic magazines?

JIM: Yes.

F. T.: Dirty magazines and masturbating and/or anything like that?

JIM: Yes.

F. T.: Do you remember doing that with friends?

JIM: On me own. Not with friends, no.

F. T.: Would that have been something you talked about with friends?

JIM: No, no, pretty embarrassing, ain't it? You know what I mean.

And later in the same interview:

F. T.: Why do you think you have attractions for women and not for men?

JIM: I don't know. I suppose because I've always been hanging around with them and what have you, I suppose. I suppose that might have something to do with it. You know, I've never really thought about it, really, to be honest.

Group differences in interviewee comfort level in talking about sexual matters should be borne in mind when considering the results presented in Chapter 6.

DATA ANALYSES

Statistical analyses with small samples present a number of problems. First, the approximation to the normal distribution required by parametric statistics is often more difficult to achieve with a small sample. For this reason, the results of the parametric analyses reported in the text were all replicated with nonparametric, or "distribution-free," tests. The small number of subjects also gives rise to the possibility that more subtle effects of the experience of growing up in a lesbian household may be overlooked, since they may fail to reach statistical significance as a result of low statistical power (the problem of Type II errors).

Although power analysis showed that for a large effect size (0.75 SD) there was an 81% chance of detecting a significant difference between groups, for a medium effect size (0.50 SD) power was only 52%. For this reason, nonsignificant trends in the data at $p < .10$ are reported in addition to the more robust findings reaching the conventional statistical significance level of $p < .05$ in a two-tailed test. We wish to emphasize, however, that the reader should be very cautious in interpreting the more tentative findings until they are replicated in other studies, particularly since the large number of statistical tests may have produced some statistically significant group differences simply by chance.

A further issue faced in the data analyses is the nonindependence of data collected from siblings (up to two children in each family could take part in the investigation). However, similar proportions of sibling pairs from each family type participated in the follow-up study, making it unlikely that the reports of siblings from any particular family could unduly influence the results. Altogether, seven pairs of siblings from lesbian mother families and five pairs of siblings from the comparison group took part in the follow-up study.

Another problem associated with small samples is the difficulty of detecting interactions between combinations of variables, for example, family type, gender, and social class. Because of the potential importance of these effects, we have attempted to address this issue. Each variable has been tested for differences between sons and daughters and for differences between children of middle- and working-class backgrounds, as well as for differences by family type. Statistically significant gender and social class differences are reported in the text, followed by an examination of possible interactions with family type.

Aside from assessing whether there were any general effects of upbringing in a lesbian household on young adults' well-being, we explored whether any particular childhood experiences were related to long-term outcomes. Longitudinal associations within the data were examined using correlations between data collected in the original study and key outcome variables assessed at follow-up. Retrospective data on the young adults' recollections of their childhood were also examined to ascertain possible associations with key outcome variables at follow-up. Again, the small sample size precluded the use of multivariate statistics. However, variables were grouped together conceptually to facilitate the understanding of the overall pattern of associations between different aspects of childhood experience and outcomes in adulthood.

The small sample size did have the advantage that an in-depth interview approach could be pursued. Verbatim transcripts were made of the interviews with young adults at follow-up. Reading and rereading these transcripts proved to be a worthwhile exercise in terms of clarifying the coding criteria applied to the interview material. The transcripts also provided valuable qualitative data in terms of the subtle meanings that may influence individual life courses. This was especially advantageous in our essentially exploratory investigation. Quotations from the transcripts have been included where these add to the interpretation of the quantitative data. The names of interviewees (and any names contained in the quotations) have all been changed to preserve confidentiality. In some cases, quotes from the same person have been attributed to different people for the same reason.

SUMMARY

In the original investigation conducted in 1976 and 1977, 27 lesbian mothers and their 39 children, as well as a comparison group of 27 heterosexual single mothers and their 39 children, participated in research interviews. The average age of the children at the time of the initial investigation was 9.5 years. For the follow-up study, carried out in 1991 and 1992, 62% of the children (8 young men and 17 young women from lesbian mother families and 12 young men and 9 young women from heterosexual mother families) were interviewed using a semistructured interview with a standardized coding scheme developed specifically for the investigation.[2] The average age of the young people interviewed at follow-up was 23.5 years.

[2]The number of respondents in the individual statistical analysis and tables presented in the following chapters may not always add up to the total number of respondents interviewed at follow-up. Particular interview ratings may not have been relevant to all respondents and occasionally there was too little information in a respondent's interview transcript to achieve a reliable rating for a particular variable.

The subsequent chapters in this book reveal what the young adults from lesbian and heterosexual mother families told us about their lives. Chapter 4 is concerned with their recollections of family life. Chapter 5 examines how the young people with lesbian mothers related to those outside their family circle, whether they presented themselves to others as coming from a lesbian mother family, how they coped with the possibility of peer prejudice, and whether their family background influenced their political attitudes. The influences of family type on sexual orientation and the formation of intimate relationships is the focus of Chapter 6. Chapter 7 assesses how young adults from both types of families fared in terms of their general well-being and adult adjustment. In the final chapter, the main findings are reviewed in the light of theoretical issues and social policy debates about lesbian and gay parenthood.

CHAPTER FOUR

Family Relationships

THE PRESENT study has provided us with the first opportunity to ask children about their mother's lesbian and heterosexual relationships. Because nearly one-third of the children with lesbian mothers in the original study were unaware of their mother's relationships, ethical considerations prevented us from raising this issue in the children's interviews. In the follow-up study we asked young adults to tell us about their family at the present time and also to reflect on what family life was like when they were growing up. Without doubt, reflections on family life are likely to be colored by current circumstances and relationships. Therefore, it is important to bear in mind that the results presented in this chapter represent the *remembered* impressions of family life as experienced by young people from lesbian or heterosexual homes.

Several issues are considered in this chapter. First, we examine whether children from lesbian mother households experience more difficult familial relationships than do children from heterosexual postdivorce families. Aspects considered here are the quality of the relationship between the child and the mother's partner, the child's impressions of the quality of the mother's relationships, and the quality of the child's relationship with both the mother and the nonresidential father. A second consideration is how aware children are of their mother's lesbian partners while they are growing up and how mothers help their children understand their relationships. Finally, we examine the variety of experiences that children have in lesbian mother families and explore which aspects influence how a young person feels about growing up in this type of family.

FAMILY RELATIONS IN LESBIAN
AND HETEROSEXUAL POSTDIVORCE FAMILIES

At the beginning of the interview the young adults were asked to give a brief description of family relationships from the time their mother and father separated. Interviewees from both lesbian and heterosexual backgrounds were asked if their mother had had any new relationships; if she had, they were asked about the new partner's gender, their own age at the time the relationship began, and whether their mother's new partner lived in the family home. This family history brought the interviewer up to date with changes in family composition since the original study and established the extent of the interviewee's knowledge of the mother's partners.

The Young Person's Relationship
with the Mother's Partner

By the time of the follow-up study, all but one of the original group of single heterosexual mothers were reported by their children to have had at least one heterosexual relationship. Furthermore, of the 20 out of 21 interviewees with heterosexual mothers who reported that their mothers had new relationships, 18 reported that the new male partner had cohabited with or married the mother. Similarly, all but one of the children with a lesbian mother remembered their mother having at least one lesbian relationship, and in 22 out of these 24 cases the mother's female partner resided with them. Therefore, in the follow-up study most young adults from both types of family could report on their experience of stepfamily relationships. Almost all (41) of the 44 young adults interviewed who reported that their mothers had a new relationship were over 10 years old at the time of their mother's main relationship (defined as the relationship remembered most clearly from the time when the participant lived at home), and in 17 cases the mother's main partner was also her current partner.

As discussed in Chapter 2, the literature on heterosexual stepfamilies emphasizes children's difficulties in adjusting to the presence of their parent's new partner, particularly with respect to a new stepmother. However, these findings are all based on heterosexual households, where the stresses and demands on step-mothers are thought to be generally greater than for stepfathers, given women's traditional responsibilities for family relationships (Visher & Visher, 1979; Ahrons & Wallisch, 1987; D. Smith, 1990). And because fathers tend to be awarded custody of children only in exceptional circumstances — such as maternal mental illness or poor predivorce mother–child relationships — stepmothers often face greater problems of integration in these homes (Clingempeel & Segal, 1986).

The situation may be very different, however, for the mother's female partner in lesbian mother families not only because the child's biological mother remains as a resident parent but also because expectations concerning the stepmother role may differ from those pertaining to heterosexual stepfamilies. Previous writing on lesbian mother families suggests that egalitarian ideals are aspired to and that co-parenting is particularly important (Blumstein & Schwartz, 1983; Dunne, 1992). However, this ideal may be more easily attained by lesbian couples who plan a family together than by those who form a stepfamily. K. G. Lewis (1980), reporting on the results of her small uncontrolled study of lesbian stepfamilies, suggests that children's difficulties with their mother's new female partner are often related to unresolved issues originating in parental divorce and to problems entailed in adjusting to stepfamily life.

In the present study, interviewees were asked how involved their mother's main partner had been in their daily welfare and whether they thought of her or him as an additional parent, a more distant family figure, or simply as their mother's partner. Interviewees were then asked to recall activities with their mother's partner and to give both positive and negative recollections of her or him. Further questioning ascertained whether the interviewees remembered any arguments with their mother's partner and the extent to which they had confided in her or him or asked for advice. This information was used to make two ratings: (1) the quality of the child's relationship with the mother's partner during adolescence and (2) the quality of the young adult's current relationship with the mother's partner. For both of these variables, ratings were made on a 4-point scale ranging from 1 (very negative) to 4 (very positive).

The results presented in Table 4.1 show that young people from lesbian mother families reported significantly better relationships both as adolescents and as adults with their mother's new female partner than did the comparison group with their mother's new male partner ($t = 2.67$, $df = 42$, $p < .05$, and $t = 3.35$, $df = 39$, $p < .01$, respectively). In addition, more than one-third of young adults from lesbian mother households (9/23) viewed their mother's main partner as an additional parent rather than as just a stepparent or their mother's girlfriend. This may reflect the closer nature of the relationship between the child and the mother's new partner in lesbian than in heterosexual households, a relationship that often involves a high level of participation in child care. In fact, in some lesbian mother households the mother's partner was reported by the young adults to have been more involved in their daily life than their mother at various times as they were growing up. For example, Megan remembered her mother's main partner in the following way:

MEGAN: I mean Sadie was like another mum really, you know, and then [when they split up] my mum gave me the opportunity to decide whether or not I wanted to stay with Sadie or with her, because you know we were just a family, you

TABLE 4.1. Quality of Young Adults' Relationships with Family Members by Family Type.

Variable	Group	Mean	SD	t	df	p
Partner–child relationship in adolescence	Lesbian mother	3.00	1.18	2.67	42	< .05
	Heterosexual mother	2.15	0.87			
Partner–young adult relationship	Lesbian mother	2.96	0.86	3.35	39	< .01
	Heterosexual mother	2.06	0.83			
Mother–young adult relationship	Lesbian mother	2.64	1.04	0.89	44	NS
	Heterosexual mother	2.38	0.92			
Father–young adult relationship	Lesbian mother	2.56	0.92	1.41	27	NS
	Heterosexual mother	2.00	1.18			

Note. From Tasker and Golombok (1995). Copyright 1995 by the American Orthopsychiatric Association, Inc. Reprinted by permission.

know. And, er, Sadie was quite prepared to just take me on if you like, because I was like her daughter, I suppose, in a way. But obviously I stayed with my mum, so even though really when I was younger I was probably closer to Sadie in a way because my mum was sort of—she's mellowed a lot with age—she was, er, um she wasn't the sort of cuddly type of person, you know. So I used to sort of ____ Sadie was the more sort of motherly sort of type. She would do all the cooking and stuff as much as I can remember, and make my clothes and all that, but I still decided to stay with my mum.

It seems that children brought up in lesbian mother households often added their mother's female partner into their family constellation as an additional family member rather than as a competitor to their absent father. In contrast, children brought up by a heterosexual mother often did not allow their mother's new male partner to become a father figure, especially if their father was still in contact with them. For example, Adrian from a heterosexual mother family said the following about the absence of a fatherly relationship with his stepfather:

ADRIAN: I mean, it's just seeing other people's family and how they are with them, just things were a bit different. I mean he wasn't really my father. I couldn't, I mean, I've related to my father, and it's a different chemistry from like relating to your father, and relating to a man that, well, he is your father, but he isn't. And there's just something different. It's hard to explain.

The Young Person's Relationship with the Mother and Father

The quality of the young adult's current relationship with their mother and father was rated separately on a 4-point scale ranging from 1 (very negative) to 4 (very positive). No differences were observed between young adults brought up by lesbian and heterosexual mothers in the quality of their current relationship with their mother (see Table 4.1). Overall, however, there was a nonsignificant trend indicating that young men tended to give more positive reports than young women of their relationship with their mother at the time of the follow-up interview ($t = 1.72, df = 44, p < .10$), just as mothers had tended to be more positive about their sons than their daughters at the time of the first study ($t = 1.68, df = 42, p < .10$). Nevertheless, no differences were found between sons from the two types of family, or between the two groups of daughters, in their rating of the quality of their relationship with their mother or their father.

In the original study, children of lesbian mothers had more regular contact with their father postseparation than did children of heterosexual mothers (Golombok et al., 1983). This group difference remained when those who did not participate in the second study were excluded from this analysis. A further indication of the absence of negative effects of being brought up by a lesbian mother on the children's relationship with their father is the finding that the groups did not differ with respect to the young adults' reports of their current relationship with their father (see Table 4.1). This variable was again rated on a 4-point scale ranging from 1 (very negative) to 4 (very positive). Both groups of young people generally reported a good relationship with their father.

Young adults were also asked about their father's attitude toward their mother's new relationship, and these reports were rated on a 3-point scale ranging from 1 (negative) to 3 (positive). Over the entire sample, young people from working-class homes reported that their father was more negative about their mother's new relationship, compared with young people from middle-class backgrounds ($t = -2.12, df = 26, p < .05$). However, there was no difference in father's attitude between young adults from lesbian and those from heterosexual mother families.

Young adults from lesbian mother families mostly reported that their father remained neutral on the topic of their mother's new girlfriend. In some cases interviewees reflected on how their not wanting to hurt their father's potentially sensitive feelings about the divorce or hear him criticize their mother prevented them from discussing this issue with him. In some cases a father might have made some initial attempt to disrupt the mother–child relationship but later gave up the attempt, as in the following example:

LIAM: From what I understand he really contested the divorce. He was very, very bad. Apparently, he tried to get Mum certified or something.

Later in the same interview Liam was asked if he and his father had ever discussed his mother's relationships with women:

LIAM: Well, we never talked about it. I don't know whether Mum ever said anything, and even though Dad knew that Mum was, you know, we had someone else living with us, I'm sure Dad must have suspected. I'm sure he must have known, but we never talked about it.

Some people recalled their father expressing a positive attitude toward their mother's new lesbian relationship, a reaction that helped them come to terms with that relationship. Helen's parents had separated when she was 5, when her mother began a lesbian relationship:

HELEN: After they'd split up, I was forever saying to my mum, "Do you think you and Dad will get back together?" And I used to go and see my dad and say, "Don't you want to get back together with my mum?" And then he just sat me down and explained it was my mum's way of living and, if so, that's fair enough. He didn't hate her or anything.

F. T.: Can you remember how old you were when your dad had these chats with you?

HELEN: Between 11 and now really. Because we still do.

LESBIAN AND HETEROSEXUAL MOTHERS' NEW RELATIONSHIPS

Mother's Relationship Style

One question that is often raised is whether lesbian mothers are more likely to have a greater number of relationships than heterosexual mothers (Blumstein & Schwartz, 1983; Kitzinger & Coyle, 1995). In the present study, the majority of lesbian mothers were no longer with the same partner they had been with at the time of the first investigation 14 years earlier. Comparable data were not available from the heterosexual mothers, who were all single at that time; however, it is known that heterosexual men and women often go through a period of experimenting with new sexual relationships after divorce (Wallerstein & Kelly, 1980). In our study it is clear from young people's reports of their mother's relationship style that there were no differences between the lesbian and the heterosexual mothers in the stability or the type of relationship that they had become involved in after the father departed (see Table 4.2). Ratings of the mother's relationship style were made on a 4-point scale ranging from 1 (one exclusive cohabiting relationship for the majority of the time) to 4 (nonexclusive relationships). Most young adults recalled their mother having either one long-term monogamous cohabiting relationship (25% of those from lesbian mother families and 35% of those from heterosexual mother families) or a series of exclusive cohabiting relationships (50% of those from lesbian mother families and 45% of those from heterosexual mother families). For example, Brendan remembered little about his mother's first two girlfriends and noticed more when his mother's girlfriend Sue moved in when he was about 10 years old.

TABLE 4.2. Young Adults' Reports of Mother's Relationships by Family Type

Variable	Group	Mean	SD	t	df	p
Mother's relationship style	Lesbian mother	3.24	1.05	1.25	44	NS
	Heterosexual mother	2.86	1.01			
Mother–partner relationship happiness	Lesbian mother	2.91	1.04	1.21	41	NS
	Heterosexual mother	2.50	1.09			
Mother–partner relationship conflict	Lesbian mother	2.59	1.05	0.42	40	NS
	Heterosexual mother	2.45	1.10			
Mother's confidant	Lesbian mother	2.44	0.95	0.20	42	NS
	Heterosexual mother	2.38	0.87			

BRENDAN: I think Sue was the first one who moved in, though not necessarily the first girlfriend, of course, and, er, Miriam, I think, came after that. And I used to quite enjoy it when Miriam was around. . . . Then Miriam left. I think Miriam and my mum weren't mentally compatible, you know.

F. T.: In what way?

BRENDAN: I don't know. I can't say that anyone was ever nasty to anyone. My mum was into different things, you know. Miriam was sort of into pop music and things like that. . . .Then there was this sort of long platonic relationship with Melissa and then there was Sara and I think that's the entire lot, really. And Sara, she's the salt-of-the-earth type; she's really, really nice. She's got a couple of kids.

Quality of Mother's Main Relationship

Conflict, rather than family structure per se, has been identified as a key factor affecting children's psychological adjustment in postdivorce families (Emery, 1982, 1988). We therefore asked interviewees to reflect on their adolescent years and to recall whether their mother had appeared to be happy in her main relationship and whether there had been either verbal or physical conflict between her and her partner. The extent of conflict in the mother's main relationship was rated on a 4-point scale with ratings ranging from 1 (regular episodes of serious conflict) to 4 (no serious conflict). Young adults' ratings of the happiness of their mother's main relationship ranged from 1 (very unhappy) to 4 (very happy over the entire relationship). No group differences were identified either for the extent of conflict between the mother and her partner or for her happiness with her partner, as reported by the young adults (see Table 4.2).

One of the main themes in the clinical literature on the effects of parental divorce on children is that under stressful conditions the child's custodial parent may be unable to function effectively in the parental role and may depend upon the child for emotional support (Minuchin, 1974; Weiss, 1979). Also of concern is whether children become involved in parental conflict

(Emery, 1988). In our study, the young adults from both lesbian and heterosexual mother families were therefore asked whether their mother had ever confided in them about relationship difficulties and whether they had ever become involved in conflict between their mother and her partner. The extent to which the child had welcomed the confidence, or felt emotionally burdened by it, was considered in rating this variable; ratings ranged from 1 (pleased that mother had confided difficulties) to 4 (felt emotionally burdened by mother's problems). The findings shown in Table 4.2 indicate that young adults from lesbian mother households in our study were no more likely to become their mother's confidant than were children of heterosexual mothers.

The following extract from Naomi's interview reflects both the closeness of her relationship with her mother, which she connects with her mother's confidences over the years, and the emotional burden of feeling desperate but powerless to help an upset parent who does not have a partner to turn to.

NAOMI: The relationship between me and my mum is obviously closer, 'cause she can confide in me. I remember one time when she was crying—and she never cries at all. And on the one hand [I did] all I could do to help her, and on the other hand I just didn't want to know. I thought I could do without this, for God's sake, I'm only 14! But then again I don't think that's 'cause my mum's a lesbian, but to do with the fact that she was on her own.

CHILDREN'S AWARENESS OF THEIR MOTHER'S LESBIAN RELATIONSHIPS

At the time of the first study only 21% (8/39) of the children of lesbian mothers were completely aware that their mother had sexual relationships with women. A further 44% (17/39) were aware that she had girlfriends, but they did not fully understand the nature of sexual relationships or that lesbian relationships are considered by society to be less acceptable than heterosexual relationships. As noted in Chapter 3, the adults who agreed to be interviewed tended to be those who as children had at least some awareness of their mother's relationships with women. By the time of the follow-up, only one child remained in ignorance of her mother's previous lesbian relationships. Therefore, the findings discussed in this book reflect the views of young people raised by lesbian mothers who were open with them about their sexual identity.

The young adults from lesbian mother families were asked when they first became aware that their mother had a romantic or sexual relationship with a woman. Most (14/24) reported a gradual awareness, with no particular incident leading to a sudden realization. Only a minority of children from lesbian mother households (7/24) remembered that their first knowledge of their mother's sexual preference was from their mother's informing them of it directly; even fewer learned of it from a particular incident (3/24). Those brought up by heterosexual mothers likewise often could not recall when they first became aware that their mother had a boyfriend (12/19).

Interviewees who had grown up in a lesbian mother family from an early age often outlined similar elements in a dawning awareness of their mother's relationships. They tended to have been initially aware that they were unlike other children in that they did not have a father, and their mother had a close relationship with a woman. They did not become aware of the sexual component until after they had begun to understand sexual relationships more generally, even though they may have seen their mother and her partner sharing a bed. In their interviews the young adults remembered that at elementary school age they had not felt uncomfortable about their mother's relationships with women and had not viewed them as being unusual. For example:

F. T.: Did you realize about them having a relationship or not?

CHERYL: Well, no, I don't think so. I mean, I don't think I was old enough to sort of, you know, to see it as a sexual relationship. She was just somebody who was around a lot, um, who was fun to be with. And she made Mum happy, I remember that as well. You know, they seemed to have a good time together, because before that Mum had been quite depressed at some points.

And later in the same interview:

F. T.: Can you remember her and Esther holding hands and kissing? [No.] No? Or Esther staying over or anything like that?

CHERYL: Well, she must have done but, you know, I can't remember ever actually sort of, you know, making a note of it. Because since then, I mean, my mum had had other relationships after that. I mean, none of them unnatural or, you know, for us to sort of think that's quite strange or anything. In fact, there was a woman who Mum had a relationship with later, who I can remember them two, those two in bed together, when we were at, um, a holiday home thing. You know, just going in to sort of talk to Mum and, you know, this woman's in bed next to her, and it, you know, that didn't mean anything, either. . . . It's just, um, you know, a natural and an expected part of her life.

In our study, a child's awareness that lesbian relationships are different from the norm often did not occur until he or she reached high school age, as in Paul's case:

F. T.: There was no sort of incident that made you think, "Oh, my Mum's got a girlfriend"?

PAUL: Well, the only thing that was an incident was when I moved on to high school [teasing by peers], and that was the time that really made me face up to my mum's going out with females, you know. Not that I thought it was terrible, but, you know, that's, that's what ____ how I became that aware that it was that different from so-called normal society, you know. But there wasn't really a first memory of thinking, "Oh no, my mum's going out with someone else, you know, a female."

In her clinical study Lewis (1980) found that children have more problems coming to terms with their mother's lesbian identity if she finds it difficult to communicate with them and answer their questions as they arise. Our interview data show that most of the children in our study felt happy with the amount they knew about their mother's relationships, and felt that she had told them neither too much nor too little. It seems that children are happiest when mothers are available to talk about issues as they occur, and do not feel comfortable when mothers give more explicit details than they want to hear. For example:

JENNY: She actually tells me more personal details, some details to do with sex and sexuality with women that she's been involved with, you know. I actually feel quite reluctant to talk to her about _____, 'cause she's quite open about like that with me and likes to talk to me, and sometimes I couldn't cope with dealing with hearing about things on such an intimate level. I'd rather not talk to her; I get all embarrassed and difficult.

Unlike Jenny, Alice was unhappy because none of her family members communicated well:

ALICE: As I said, from a young age ____ I can remember at a young age knowing what was going on, but no one would talk to me about it. . . . I think perhaps the only thing I wish was that perhaps that we were a bit more open.

F. T.: Told you a bit more?

ALICE: Talked a bit more. You know, asked me, talked to me, instead of getting on and doing it.

All interviewees were asked how open their mother had been in showing physical affection to her female or male partner and whether they had felt embarrassed about this at the time. Children of lesbian mothers were no more likely than children of heterosexual mothers to report feeling unhappy or embarrassed about their mother being physically affectionate to her partner in front of them (7/19 children of lesbian mothers felt their mother had been too open about her physical relationship, as did 4/17 children of heterosexual mothers). None of the children first discovered their mother's lesbian identity through seeing her engaged in sexual intimacy with her partner. One child found out about her mother's lesbian feelings by inadvertently observing her mother and her partner kissing; there is no evidence that this event presented a problem for her, possibly because her mother talked to her about it immediately afterward.

YOUNG PEOPLE'S ATTITUDES
TOWARD THEIR NONTRADITIONAL FAMILY

Following up in early adulthood a sample of children brought up by lesbian and heterosexual mothers has provided us with an opportunity to systematically assess children's feelings about their mother's sexual identity. Previous uncontrolled studies of children raised by lesbian mothers suggest that children may have problems initially in accepting their mother's lesbian identity (K. G. Lewis, 1980), particularly in the case of older adolescent boys (Hall, 1978; K. G. Lewis, 1980). However, it has been suggested that young people may be more accepting of their mother's sexual orientation if they learn of it early in childhood (Pennington, 1987; Huggins, 1989). Huggins reported that girls from single-parent lesbian mother families tend to have lower self-esteem than those who live with their mother and her female partner and that adolescent girls from lesbian single-parent families and stepfamilies have a more positive self-concept if family relationships are good and if the responses of others outside the family (including their father) are not hostile to the new family setup. It has also been proposed that children of lesbians fare best in homes where the mother has a strong positive identity and good parenting skills and is well integrated into a supportive social network that includes other lesbian mother families (Pennington, 1987). Furthermore, a study of the well-being of lesbian mothers themselves found that those who are "out" about their sexual identity tend to have higher self-esteem and that their psychological health is positively associated with involvement in the lesbian community and feminist politics (Rand, Graham, & Rawlings, 1982).

On the other hand, public concern is often expressed that children may be more likely to be stigmatized by peers if their mother is open about being lesbian and active in lesbian politics ("B v B," 1991). School-age children in K. G. Lewis's (1980) study reported that they often worried about being teased or ostracized by their peers and that this affected how they felt about their mother's relationships. The potentially hostile response of peers to children growing up in lesbian mother families is, not surprisingly, also of major concern to lesbian mothers themselves (Lesbian Mothers Group, 1989).

Most of the children of lesbian mothers in Lewis's study came to admire their mother for her stance against convention. However, in her journal article Lewis juxtaposes children's intellectual acceptance of their mother's right to express her sexual preference with the continued ambivalence on the part of some children toward their mother's identity, an ambivalence that finds expression in the child's disproportionate fear of social stigma, intense anger at a particular aspect of household arrangements, reluctance to discuss negative incidents, or tendency to act out feelings through such behaviors as leaving home.

In the present study, a 4-point rating scale of the young person's feelings about his or her nontraditional family identity was constructed on the basis of Lewis's typology; interviewees were classified as feeling 1 (resentful), 2 (embarrassed), 3 (accepting), or 4 (proud of their family identity). Young adults in the heterosexual mother control group were also rated on this scale with respect to their feelings concerning their mother's identity as a nonmarried heterosexual woman. Ratings were made both for interviewees feelings while in high school and as young adults. Data relating to the quality of the relationship between the young person and the mother's partner were excluded from these ratings.

No group differences were found for young adults' retrospective reports of how they had felt as adolescents about their mother's relationships, that is, with a female partner in the case of lesbian mothers and with a male partner who was not their father in the case of heterosexual mothers (see Table 4.3). Thirty-eight percent (9/24) of young adults from lesbian backgrounds felt that they had accepted their mother's having lesbian relationships and reported that they had not attempted to keep their family identity secret from close friends at school, 33% (8/24) had felt embarrassed during adolescence about coming from a lesbian mother family, and 29% (7/24) had opposed their mother over this issue. Within the lesbian mother group, no gender or

TABLE 4.3. Young Adults' Reports of Their Own Feelings and
Their Mothers' Feelings about Their Mother's Identity, by Family Type

Variable	Group	Mean	SD	t	df	p
Adolescent feelings about family identity	Lesbian mother	2.08	0.83	-1.41	42	NS
	Heterosexual mother	2.45	0.89			
Adult feelings about family identity	Lesbian mother	3.21	0.78	2.11	41	$< .05$
	Heterosexual mother	2.74	0.65			
Young adult's report of mother's happiness with her identity	Lesbian mother	2.39	0.66	2.70	42	$< .01$
	Heterosexual mother	1.86	0.66			

Note. From Tasker and Golombok (1995). Copyright 1995 by the American Orthopsychiatric Association, Inc. Reprinted by permission.

social class differences were found with regard to acceptance/rejection of family identity during adolescence.

As young adults, those brought up by lesbian mothers were significantly more positive about their family identity than were those raised by the comparison group of heterosexual mothers ($t = 2.11, df = 41, p < .05$; see Table 4.3). For the young adults within the lesbian mother group, no gender or social class differences were found with respect to feelings about their family identity. The results of paired t tests comparing changes in feelings about family identity between adolescence and young adulthood showed that children from lesbian mother families became more positive about their upbringing in a nontraditional household ($t = -5.82, df = 23, p < .001$). There was also a nonsignificant trend toward more positive attitudes among children from heterosexual mother families ($t = -1.76, df = 17, p < .10$).

As young adults, 38% (9/24) of those who had been brought up by lesbian mothers were proud of their mother's sexual identity and were open to acquaintances about her lesbian relationships, and 50% (12/24) were accepting of their mother's having lesbian relationships. Although 84% (16/19) of the children of heterosexual mothers accepted their mother's identity as a single parent with a boyfriend or as a remarried mother and were happy to talk about this with friends, none thought of it as an issue they would be proud to discuss with acquaintances. Children from lesbian backgrounds who were proud of their mother's identity often saw this as a political matter and sought to inform public opinion on gay rights by giving their own family history. This was true in Bob's case:

BOB: I mean I use it as a riposte when you get people in the pub being antigay or whatever or talking about benders and what have you. I bring it out selectively then, you know (*laugh*).

F. T.: Are there occasions when you wouldn't say something?

BOB: Oh well, no, no only in the—well, you just have to choose who you would maybe want to start an argument with about the matter. It's only in that sort of way, you know. If it was a very large and drunken bloke, then you probably wouldn't . . . but if it's just my workmates . . . , because none of my friends would fall into that category. But with workmates and stuff, if they make casual remarks often in work or after work, then I pick them up on it.

In contrast, the young adults from nontraditional heterosexual backgrounds were more likely to view their mother's lifestyle as her personal choice and the details of this as a private, family matter.

F. T.: What about people you meet now? I mean, would you tell them about your family?

MARK: No. Only my wife. But apart from that, no like, you know.

F. T.: Is there any reason why you wouldn't tell them about your family?

MARK: I suppose because it's none of their business, basically. I wouldn't like to say, because I've never been in that situation to, you know, say that he's [my stepdad] and he ain't [my dad] type of thing. You know what I mean.

Interviewees were also asked how positive they thought their mother was about her identity as a lesbian or as a nonmarried heterosexual woman (rated on a 3-point scale ranging from 1, negative to 3, positive). Forty-eight percent (11/23) of young adults from lesbian mother households considered their mother to be positive about her lesbian identity; only two interviewees thought that she considered her sexual identity to be without any advantages. Children brought up by nonmarried heterosexual mothers were more likely to report that their mother was negative about her nontraditional identity and preferred to be married ($t = 2.70$, $df = 42$, $p < .01$; see Table 4.3).

ACCEPTANCE OF FAMILY IDENTITY DURING ADOLESCENCE AND ADULTHOOD AMONG YOUNG ADULTS BROUGHT UP BY A LESBIAN MOTHER

For participants from lesbian mother families, Pearson product–moment correlation coefficients were calculated between each of the two dependent variables (acceptance of family identity in adolescence and acceptance of family identity in adulthood) and variables from both the initial study (see Table 4.4) and the follow-up study (see Table 4.5).[1] Owing to the small sample size, correlation coefficients with p values of less than .10 are reported; these should be interpreted with caution. From the existing literature, it was expected that acceptance of family identity would be associated with positive and stable family relationships, the father's acceptance of the new family structure, the mother's acceptance of her lesbian identity, the mother's discretion in relating to others outside the family (particularly with respect to the child's friends), and the absence of stigmatization from the peer group.

Acceptance of Family Identity during Adolescence

Only one variable from the initial study was significantly correlated with feelings during the high school years about coming

---

[1]A similar set of investigations was attempted on the data from young adults brought up by heterosexual mothers. However, as there was little variation among this group of young people in terms of their acceptance of family identity, further analyses were abandoned.

TABLE 4.4. Correlations between Childhood Family Characteristics at the Time of the Initial Study and Acceptance of Family Identity in Adolescence and in Adulthood

	Acceptance in adolescence	Acceptance in adulthood
Family relationships at time of initial study		
Mother's expressed warmth to child (0, "none"–5, "very warm")	−.214 (23)	−.182 (23)
Mother's relationship history (0, "four partners or fewer"–1, "more than four partners or concurrent relationships")	−.415* (24)	.347† (24)
Quality of mother's relationship with her female partner (1, "fully harmonious"–5, "serious conflict")	.128 (13)	.224 (13)
Mother and partner share child care (0, "mother and partner share"–1, "mother main caregiver")	.128 (13)	.416 (13)
Child's contact with father (0, "none"–2, "at least weekly")	−.190 (24)	.222 (24)
Number of years child raised in heterosexual home	.116 (24)	.044 (24)
Child's awareness of mother's lesbian identity (0, "none"–2, "fully aware")	.204 (24)	.059 (24)
Mother's identity at time of initial study		
Mother's contentment with her sexual identity (1, "prefer to be heterosexual"–5, "positive about lesbian identity")	−.020 (24)	−.270 (24)
Mother's political involvement (0, "no involvement in lesbian/gay politics"–3, "frequent involvement")	−.183 (24)	.044 (24)
Mother's openness about lesbian identity at time of initial study		
Mother's openness in showing affection in front of child (0, "none"–2, "kiss/caress")	−.189 (18)	.358 (18)
Mother "out" in local community (0, "no"–2, "public knowledge")	.050 (24)	.133 (24)
Mother "out" to child's school teachers (0, "no"–2, "discussed with teachers")	−.068 (24)	.400† (24)
Mother's attitude toward men (1, "negative"–5, "some sexual feelings toward men")	−.086 (24)	−.018 (24)

(*continued*)

TABLE 4.4. *cont.*

	Acceptance in adolescence	Acceptance in adulthood
Peers' response at time of initial study		
Quality of child's peer relationships (0, "good"–2, "definite difficulties")	.239 (18)	.331 (18)

† $p < .10$; * $p < .05$.

from a lesbian mother family. Young adults whose mothers reported a relationship history of short-term relationships or affairs were more likely than other young adults from lesbian mother families to be negative about their family identity during adolescence ($r = -0.415$, $p < .05$; see Table 4.4). Similarly, we found that the equivalent variable, mother's relationship style, assessed retrospectively in the follow-up study, was associated with more negative feelings during adolescence about the mother's lesbian identity ($r = -.662$, $p < .001$; see Table 4.5). A possible explanation is that mothers who have a number of relationships appear more openly lesbian and thus raise the issue of their lifestyle in a more direct way than do mothers who have a long-term relationship with one partner. Furthermore, it has been observed that children in postdivorce families can be extremely upset when their mother or father experiments with a series of new heterosexual relationships (Wallerstein & Blakeslee, 1989).

Two other variables measuring family relationships at follow-up were associated with young adults' retrospective reports of acceptance of their family during adolescence (see Table 4.5). Young adults who felt closer to their mother reported greater acceptance of their family identity as adolescents ($r = .503$, $p < .05$), and there was a nonsignificant trend suggesting that those who described a good relationship with their mother's current partner also reported greater acceptance of coming from a lesbian mother family as an adolescent ($r = .371$, $p < .10$). Adolescents who felt most positively about their mother's identity may have developed closer relationships with their mother and her partner. Alternatively, those who had closer relationships in adulthood may have forgotten any earlier difficulties.

TABLE 4.5. Correlations between Family Characteristics Reported at Follow-Up and Acceptance of Family Identity in Adolescence and in Adulthood

	Acceptance in adolescence	Acceptance in adulthood
Family relationships at follow-up		
Current relationship with mother (1, "very negative"–4, "very positive")	.503* (24)	.305 (24)
Adolescent relationship with mother's partner (1, "very negative"–4, "very positive")	.311 (24)	.142 (24)
Current relationship with mother's partner (1, "very negative"–4, "very positive")	.371† (24)	–.117 (24)
Mother's relationship style (1, "exclusive"–4, "nonexclusive")	–.662*** (24)	–.002 (24)
Mother's satisfaction with primary relationship (1, "very unhappy"–4, "very happy")	.005 (23)	–.141 (23)
Conflict in mother's primary relationship (1, "regular episodes of conflict"– 4, "no serious conflict")	.046 (22)	–.220 (22)
Closeness of current relationship with father (1, "very negative"–4, "very positive")	.064 (18)	–.064 (18)
Father's attitude toward mother's relationship (1, "opposed/upset"–3, "expressed support")	.196 (17)	.030 (17)
Mother's identity at follow-up		
Mother's contentment with her identity (1, "prefer to be heterosexual"–3, "very positive")	–.285 (23)	–.170 (23)
Mother's involvement in feminist politics (0, "not involved"–1, "feminist")	–.164 (23)	.380† (23)
Mother's involvement in lesbian/gay rights politics (0, "not involved"–1, "involvement")	.052 (23)	.380† (23)
Mother's openness about lesbian identity and attitude toward child's friends at follow-up		
Mother's openness in showing physical affection in front of child (0, "interviewee not embarrassed"–1, "some embarrassment felt")	–.412† (19)	.070 (19)
Mother's openness about her lifestyle in front of school friends (0, "discrete"–1, "too open")	–.596** (23)	–.110 (23)
Mother's response to school friends visiting home (1, "very unwelcoming"–3, "welcoming")	.402† (24)	.181 (24)

(continued)

TABLE 4.5. *cont.*

	Acceptance in adolescence	Acceptance in adulthood
Mother's response to young adult's own relationship partners (1, "disapproving"– 3, "welcoming")	.547** (24)	.106 (24)
Mother's attitude toward men (0, "negative"–1, "neutral or positive")	.428† (21)	.229 (21)
Peers' response at follow-up		
Teased about mother's lifestyle (0, "not teased"–1, "teased about mother")	– .397† (24)	– .099 (24)
Teased about own sexuality (0, "not teased"–1, "teased about sexuality")	– .609** (24)	– .361† (24)

† $p < .10$; * $p < .05$; ** $p < .01$; *** $p < .001$.

In our study neither the quality of the mother's primary relationship nor the quality of the children's relationship with their mother's partner during their adolescent years appeared to be central to how the children felt about having a lesbian mother. Children who had a poor relationship with their mother's partner during adolescence could still feel positively about coming from a lesbian mother family. Conversely, one of the few participants who was extremely negative about having a lesbian mother had experienced fairly good relationships with all of her mother's female partners (in contrast to her stormy relationship with her mother). Part of the reason for Sharon's poor relationship with her mother seems to relate to her mother's openness about her relationships with women and the embarrassment Sharon felt about this (a point that we shall return to later):

SHARON: I like June because she was sort of like a closet gay. She didn't like walking around with Mum hand in hand, whereas her and Marie do, and that embarrasses me. I hated that. 'Cause my mum did quite a few embarrassing things to me when I were in my teenage way.

Uncontrolled studies have found that the extent to which children have come to terms with their parents' divorce is a key factor in determining their willingness to accept their mother's lesbian identity (K. G. Lewis, 1980). However, there were few indications of resentment of the divorce from the interviewees in the present study, perhaps because of the length of time that had elapsed since the divorce. Contrary to the findings of Huggins (1989), there is no general evidence from this study that the father's opposition or support for the mother's lesbian relationship influences a child's acceptance or rejection of the mother's lesbian identity. As mentioned previously, young adults in this study often did not discuss their mother's relationships with their father, and if they did so, they were not necessarily swayed by his opinions.

The negative response of peers during high school as recollected at follow-up also appeared to be strongly associated with a more negative view of family identity during adolescence (see Table 4.5). Young people who recalled being teased about their own sexuality reported less acceptance of their family identity during their high school years ($r = -.609$, $p < .01$). A nonsignificant trend also suggested that interviewees who reported being teased about their mother's lifestyle tended to recall feeling less positive about their family identity during adolescence ($r = -.397$, $p < .10$). The negative response of others, therefore, may have a corresponding negative effect on a child's own attitudes toward his or her family. Melanie's feelings when she first knew about her mother's lesbian relationship were influenced by her concerns about being ostracized by her peers and the comments of their parents:

F. T.: How did you feel about your mother being a lesbian when you first knew?

MELANIE: It hurt. It hurt me.

F. T.: Why did you feel like that?

MELANIE: Well, my mum were different to everybody else's mum, I suppose. I never had a dad, and I were always going to have a woman living there, who we didn't particularly know. But I think it were more my pride. I'd got all my friends to find out, and it worked out that my friends didn't want to know me. I mean, it didn't bother my mum that I had no friends. I mean, people would talk to me, but as for going home with me . . . And then there were their parents saying, "You're not going to Melanie's house. Her mother's funny." Things like that. That's how I lost my friends, 'cause of their parents.

Congruent with these findings, a number of follow-up study variables relating to whether or not the young adults felt their mother had been too open about her lesbian relationships were found to significantly correlate with young adults' lower acceptance of their family identity during adolescence. Those who felt that their mother had been too open about her lifestyle in front of their school friends were more likely to report that they had had negative feelings about their family identity during their high school years ($r = -.596, p < .01$). The results in Table 4.5 also show a nonsignificant trend suggesting that those who had felt embarrassed about their mother showing affection to her partner tended to have been less accepting of their family during adolescence ($r = -412, p < .10$).

In contrast, young people who felt their mother was sensitive to their need for discretion felt more positive about their family identity, perhaps because they were reassured that only trusted friends would learn about their family background. This finding is in line with that of Bozett (1988), who in his research on children of gay fathers highlighted the importance for young people of feeling in control of the information peers receive about their family circumstances.

There was also a nonsignificant trend in our data suggesting that young adults reported having had more positive feelings during adolescence about coming from a lesbian mother family if their mother had welcomed school friends' visits to their home ($r = .402, p < .10$). In addition, those who felt their mother had been accepting of their own boyfriends or girlfriends were more likely to have held a favorable view of their family identity ($r = .547, p < .01$). Young adults who reported that their mother held a positive view of men also tended to have been more accepting of their family identity during adolescence, although this association failed to reach statistical significance ($r = .428, p < .10$). Since young people who felt their mother welcomed their own partner also reported that their mother had a more positive attitude toward men ($r = -.472, p < .05$), a link is suggested between these two variables and acceptance of their family identity for a sample composed mostly of girls, the majority of whom had heterosexual relationships during adolescence. For example, Rosie felt positive about her mother's lesbian identity and talked about how all her friends used to meet at her house before going out to a nightclub.

ROSIE: Yeah, my friends got on really well with my mum, and they all came round. . . . And my friends brought their boyfriends round to meet up before we went out anywhere.

It is interesting to note that neither the child's gender, the socioeconomic status of the family, nor the child's age when the mother identified herself as lesbian were significantly associated with feelings about the mother's lesbian identity. This suggests that these variables are less important than the mother's sensitivity to the situation and how peers outside the family respond. However, the small sample size may have resulted in more subtle effects remaining undetected.

Acceptance of Family Identity in Adulthood

When the variables associated with interviewees' feelings in adulthood about their mother's identity are examined, the picture changes. The majority of the variables that were found to relate to acceptance or rejection of the mother's lesbian identity during adolescence were not found to significantly relate to young adults' current feelings about their mother's identity. However, the association between memories of having been teased about their own sexuality during their school days and feeling opposed to or embarrassed about coming from a lesbian mother family remained as a nonsignificant trend ($r = -.361, p < .10$).

The results in Table 4.4 also show a nonsignificant trend suggesting that the young people who were most positive about their family identity tended to have mothers who were open about their lesbian identity to their child's school at the time of the first study ($r = .400, p < .10$). Also, those whose mothers reported having a greater number of relationships prior to the original study tended to have a more positive view of their family identity as young adults ($r = .347, p < .10$).

Whether or not their mother was politically active made no difference to the young person's acceptance or rejection of their family background during their adolescent years. Nevertheless, there were nonsignificant trends in the data suggesting that those whose mother had been involved in the gay rights movement tended to be more positive about their family identity in adulthood ($r = .380, p < .10$), as did those who reported that their mother had been involved in feminist politics ($r = .380, p < .10$). This again suggests an association between open and positive attitudes toward lesbian issues on the part of the mother and greater acceptance by young adults of their family identity.

Finally, a caveat about the interpretation of these results: Since most of the variables found to be significantly correlated with adolescent and adult feelings about coming from a lesbian mother family are measures taken from the follow-up study, causality cannot be presumed and interpretations must be treated as suggestive rather than definitive. Only one variable (the number of relationships the mother had experienced) had any significant prospective association at the 5% level with how sons or daughters felt about their family identity during their adolescent years.

SUMMARY

In general, the children in our study who had grown up in lesbian mother households were positive about their family life. Young adults from lesbian mother families gave more positive accounts of their relationship with their mother's female partner than did those in the comparison group in relation to stepfathers. A mother's female partner could perhaps more easily fit into the role of a "second mum." Thus, these findings relating to children's perceptions of lesbian postdivorce families challenge the conclusions drawn from previous research on heterosexual stepfamilies concerning the difficulties of stepmother–stepchild relationships.

In their reflections on their feelings during adolescence, those young adults from lesbian mother families were on average no more negative about their family identity than were those from heterosexual mother families. Young adults who did describe adolescent feelings of opposition or embarrassment about having a lesbian mother were those who also reported that their mother had not accepted their own partners, those who had a poor relationship with their mother currently, and those whose mother had become involved in more short-term relationships. Furthermore, adolescent difficulties in coming to terms with having a lesbian mother were particularly associated with being teased at school about one's own sexuality and were compounded if the child felt that the mother had not been aware of or sympathetic to this. How children from lesbian mother families dealt with friends' reactions will be discussed further in the next chapter.

By early adulthood the young men and women in our study who were brought up in lesbian postdivorce families generally were more positive about their family identity than were those brought up in heterosexual postdivorce families. Those whose mothers had been open about their lesbian identity and were active in feminist or lesbian and gay politics showed a tendency toward greater pride in their family of origin.

CHAPTER FIVE

The Family and
the Outside World

A MAJOR challenge for every child and his or her family is the integration of family experience with the wider society outside the home. Although a universal issue, integration is potentially more difficult to achieve the greater the family's divergence from prevailing norms within the wider social group (Berg, 1985). This chapter is concerned with how children from lesbian mother families respond to differences between their family background and the dominant heterosexual culture in which they grow up. Until recently, the predominant view was that children with lesbian or gay parents would be disadvantaged in their relationships outside the family by the prejudice they would face from some heterosexual men and women. However, recent commentators have suggested that children brought up by lesbian or gay parents may benefit from their personal experience of diversity within a community and may therefore be less restricted in their outlook and more able to appreciate today's multicultural society (Patterson, 1992). First, we consider to what extent children from lesbian mother families are able to integrate their friends with family life. We then examine whether children from lesbian mother families are stigmatized in school because of their family background. Finally, we explore whether children from lesbian mother families have a more positive attitude toward gay and lesbian rights within society and a more sympathetic attitude toward feminist issues.

INTEGRATION OF FAMILY AND FRIENDS

Bozett (1987, 1988) has described some strategies used by children of gay fathers to successfully manage potential difficulties with peer prejudice. It is often possible for such children to prevent their father's sexual identity from becoming widely known by maintaining a boundary between their family and their peers. Alternatively, in order to preempt a negative reaction, children may decide to selectively tell others that their father is gay.

Telling Friends

In the present study, young adults from lesbian mother families were asked whether school friends had been aware of their mother's lesbian identity and, if so, how they had learned of it. Interviewees were categorized as follows: 1 (friends did not know), 2 (friends had found out), 3 (friends were assumed to have known because the family identity was obvious), or 4 (friends were told by the young person). Table 5.1 shows the number of young adults in lesbian mother families whose school friends were aware of their mother's lesbian identity. The majority of interviewees appear to have been in control of the information that friends were given about their mother's identity. Fourteen (61%) had felt comfortable enough to disclose that they had a lesbian mother to at least one close friend, either by telling the friend directly or by not hiding their mother's lesbian lifestyle. Nine (39%) had decided not to disclose any information concerning their mother's sexual identity to any of their school friends. In five of these cases friends remained unaware of the adolescent's family background. Only four interviewees reported that friends (or friends' parents) had found out about their family background when they did not want them to know.

We also asked about friends' responses to learning about the interviewee's family background. Responses relating to this variable were rated as 1 (all friends negative), 2 (at least one friend negative at first), 3 (friends neutral or accepting), or 4 (friends positive). Of the 18 interviewees whose friends knew about their mother's lesbian identity, five had met with a negative response from friends, although in two cases the friends later became more positive (see Table 5.1).

TABLE 5.1. School Friends' Awareness of and Response to Family Background

	School friends' awareness			
	Friends did not know	Friends found out	Friends probably knew	Friends told
Young adults from lesbian mother families	5 (22%)	4 (17%)	4 (17%)	10 (44%)

	School friends' response			
	Friends negative	Friends initially negative	Friends accepting	Friends positive
Young adults from lesbian mother families	3 (17%)	2 (11%)	10 (55%)	3 (17%)

Feeling different from friends and deciding what to tell friends about their family were major concerns for some children from lesbian mother families. As Judith said:

JUDITH: I sort of felt sometimes like "Why can't she just be like other mums? Why can't we just be like other families." You know. I remember, you know, feeling that. And there were times when I felt like it was fine, you know. But when she was open about it in public, I felt that she was being too open, because none of my friends at school had mums who were going out with ladies and it was just like for my friendships, because I wanted to be friends with other kids. . . . It was affecting it in a dramatic way, not necessarily the fact that she was with women. But if she wasn't with women, then she was with a younger bloke, or she was not conforming in some other way. . . . And I thought, that's fine; it's fine for you to have your own life and do your own things, but I sort of resented the fact that it affected what other kids, or what their parents, would say.

Young adults from single-parent heterosexual backgrounds were asked similar questions about how they handled telling friends about their family background. All had told at least one friend about their mother being a single parent who had a boyfriend, and in all cases their friends had been accepting. Many interviewees from heterosexual mother families said that they knew others in their class who were in similar family circumstances:

F. T.: Were you ever concerned to keep things quiet about what was happening at home with your mum because it might be difficult at school?

MICHAEL: Well, it was something I didn't put a great deal of thought into because quite a number of my friends did have single parents. So not that I saw that I stood out any different from them. I know that a couple of them, I didn't go round there and see any boyfriends, for instance, but, um, you know, I just assumed that they may have a boyfriend like my mum. Like my friend Dave, for instance. He used to say, "My mum went out to dinner last night with such and such." . . . You know that someone's mum is going to be seeing other men. It was open really, like accepted. It wasn't something that I saw that was out of the ordinary.

The potential for attracting social stigma varies according to the degree to which the family group contravenes the social norm of the heterosexual nuclear family. Therefore, the implications of their mother's new relationship for attracting peer prejudice differed for children from lesbian versus heterosexual backgrounds. The visibility of the household as a nontraditional family increased when a lesbian mother and her female partner decided to make a home together. In contrast, when single heterosexual mothers married, or had a new male partner move into the home, the new household unit came closer to the nuclear family norm. The social implications were therefore very different from these associated with a new lesbian partnership, as can be seen in this extract from Nigel's interview:

F. T.: Did the issue of your mum and Pete having married come up at all at school? I mean, did the teachers know anything about it?

NIGEL: Yeah, because I think I was proud at the time that I had a father figure now. I'd say, "I've got a stepfather," and they'd go, "Ooh, he's got a stepfather." And when they got married, it was like I was very happy.

F. T.: So friends that you had, they all knew about it, and it wasn't a difficult thing to tell them?

NIGEL: I think it was amazement to them: "Ooh, stepfather! Ooh!" You know? Because they had fathers, you know, "Who's your dad then? Who's your real dad?" And that . . . I think as a young child I didn't really know who my dad was, you know. But all I knew now was that I had a new one.

Many of the young adults from lesbian mother families knew no other children approximately their age who were also growing up in a lesbian mother family (although systematic data were not collected on this topic). However, nearly all of the young adults interviewed remembered at least one school friend whose mother and father had separated. Therefore, their experience of living in a father-absent household was not so unusual, particularly when their mother did not have a partner living at home. Despite this, many of the children from lesbian mother families recalled feeling isolated from others for at least part of their school years. As Beverly said:

BEVERLY: I mean, I never knew if there was anybody else going through the same thing at school. But I've said to [my sister] quite a few times [that] I wish I could have known if anybody else's parents were gay, 'cause at least then you could, like, talk about it, and see if they were going through the same thing.

Bringing Friends Home

We examined the extent to which interviewees recalled maintaining a boundary between their school life and their home life in order to prevent peers from making the discovery that they came from a lesbian mother family. The inability to invite school friends home, either because of their own embarrassment or because of their mother's discouragement of such behavior, was perhaps the clearest indication that they wished to keep friends and family separate. It was not the case that interviewees from lesbian mother families found it more difficult to bring friends home than did young people from heterosexual backgrounds. As shown in Table 5.2, no significant difference was found between young adults from the two types of family regarding how welcoming their mother (or her partner) had been to their friends.

Bozett (1988) identified four factors that are likely to influence how young people feel about allowing others outside the family to know about their gay father: the age or maturity of the child, mutuality (the extent to which the child identifies with the parent's differentness), the family's living arrangements, and how obvious or obtrusive the parent's sexual identity is perceived to be. Our interview data suggest that young people's age and the extent to which they want to assert their individuality appear to influence how open about their family background they are prepared to be. The following extract from Kim's interview shows that for older adolescents a degree of prestige can be attached to coming from a lesbian mother family if the circumstances are favorable:

KIM: I set up this sixth-form discussion group about sexual differences and heterosexuality and homosexuality. . . . It was a bit sort of "Hey, look at me!" I know all about this when everybody is leading normal little sheltered schoolgirl lives. It was sort of it gave me a bit of something, a bit of social standing I suppose.

TABLE 5.2. Mother's Response to Young Person's School Friends by Family Type

	Lesbian mother	Heterosexual mother	Fisher's exact p
Mother always welcoming to adolescent's friends	12	10	NS
Occasionally difficult to bring friends home	7	9	
Always difficult to bring friends home	6	2	

Note. Fisher's exact test p calculated for "mother always welcoming to adolescent's friends" versus "occasionally/always difficult to bring friends home."

However, as Peter's example (below) indicates, the decision of whether to maintain a boundary between home and school is also influenced by the adolescent's judgment of peers' maturity and the general acceptance of gay men and lesbian women:

F. T.: Did you bring high school friends home at all?

PETER: When I really started bringing friends home was towards the end of the sixth form. Everyone was a bit more mature and everyone was more able to handle things like this, things like my mum's a lesbian, and, you know, it was easier to talk about. But not before then usually, no; not as a conscious decision. It just didn't really come up to, like, take them home.

F. T.: What about when you were in [elementary] school, can you remember bringing friends home then?

PETER: I know I had friends home, but as far as I know, my mother was the normal act — you know, like "I'm not a lesbian, I'm just a mother," which meant that any friends that came over just saw the mother side.

Living arrangements also affected how easy it was for interviewees to bring friends home. Living in a relatively large house meant, for some children, that when they brought their friends home with them, there was little contact between their friend's and their parents. However, for Wendy, as for other young people, the practicalities of household space meant that privacy was a major issue:

F. T.: So did you bring friends home at all, or was that difficult?

WENDY: It was slightly difficult 'cause of the flat, yeah, but I did get them round a couple of times when my mum was out. . . . But it was only when I got to college, really — after school, when I was 16 or 17 — that I met two people there, a gay bloke and a black woman . . . that I did actually talk to them about it, you know. And they met her. . . . I just remember it being difficult about bringing people home slightly, not necessarily because my mum was a lesbian or she was with another woman but more to do with the [small] flat and that I didn't have a room that was closed off from the rest of the flat.

How visible young people feel their mother's lesbian identity is to other people may, for some, be a major determinant of how comfortable they are in allowing friends to meet their family. According to Bozett (1988), whether or not a young person feels that the parent's homosexual identity is obvious, or obtrusive, is likely to hinge on the extent to which the parent conforms to stereotypical images of gay or lesbian behavior, or displays symbols proclaiming a gay or lesbian identity. The fear of attracting prejudice meant that some young people in our study had worried during adolescence about others finding out about their lesbian mother and had felt concerned that her lesbian identity was obvious to friends, for instance, through lesbian or feminist badges, posters, or books around the home or through her affectionate behavior toward her girlfriend. In most cases, the young people's feeling that their mother had been indiscreet probably reflected their own sensitivity to her lesbian identity, together with their fear of prejudice, and not a deliberate, or even unintentional, act on their mother's part that resulted in her informing others. As Goffman (1963) indicated, it is the potential for being discredited, and the perceived visibility of the source of stigma, that is most relevant when considering a young person's response to the impulse to invite friends home:

F. T.: What about bringing friends home?

JEROME: We'd always be round at each other's houses, mainly at Pete and Linda's. They'd come round here from time to time. . . . Sometimes there'd be a poster up or something and I'd be a bit concerned about it and have to get them into my room before they saw it or I'd hope they wouldn't see it or I'd have to hide it or something. But they either didn't see it or else they never commented on it, because nobody ever said anything about it, anyway.

Interviewees from lesbian mother families who had brought friends home during their adolescence were asked whether they felt that their mother had been too open about her lesbian identity. About one-third (9/23) felt that their mother had not been as discreet in front of their school friends as they would have liked. It was not meaningful to ask the equivalent question of interviewees from heterosexual backgrounds. As is clear from Michael's comment, presented earlier, a mother's heterosexual relationships were not kept secret from school friends by our interviewees because her identity as a single or partnered but unmarried heterosexual mother did not carry social stigma; furthermore, heterosexual mothers could be more intimate with their male partner, for example, in holding hands, without their son or daughter feeling embarrassed in front of friends.

The young people in our study who had a lesbian mother seemed to feel most comfortable with bringing friends home when their mother was sensitive to the possibility that her being too open might lead to later prejudice against and difficulties for her child. Bozett (1988) reported that children of gay fathers sometimes modify their own behavior, or try to control their father's behavior, so that friends will not become aware of their parent's gay identity. However, in our study the mothers themselves were generally highly tuned to possible occasions for other people's prejudice and assiduously avoided any show of affection to their partner or any reference to lesbian issues when their son or daughter had company. As Geraldine said:

F. T.: Did you ever feel that Lynne or your mum were too open with the school, with teachers, or with friends?

GERALDINE: No. No, not at all.

F. T.: Or had books?

GERALDINE: They always keep the books on the bottom shelf behind the television. Therefore unless somebody's actually looking at the book shelves, they'd never see the books. There's never been any evidence of it.

F. T.: Posters or badges?

GERALDINE: No, no there's never been any evidence of it. You know, apart from in the home they'd never hold hands or kiss on the cheek and what have you, and they would never have dreamed of doing that in front of people I'd brought back.

PEER PREJUDICE

One of the objections to granting lesbian mothers custody of their children that is invariably raised during custody proceedings is that the children will be teased about their mother's sexual orientation and ostracized by their peers. Concern that their children may experience prejudice because of their sexual identity is also a major topic of discussion among lesbian mothers themselves (Lesbian Mothers Group, 1989).

In our initial study in 1976–1977, mothers were asked about their children's friendships and popularity with peers. No differences in quality of friendships were identified between children raised in lesbian mother families and those raised in heterosexual mother families. Similarly, in the investigation by Green et al. (1986) no differences between children brought up by lesbian mothers and those raised by heterosexual mothers were found for the children's perceptions of their popularity with peers or for mother-rated measures of the children's sociability and social acceptance. It seems, therefore, that younger children in lesbian mother families generally do not encounter problems with their wider peer group.

Nevertheless, it is often argued that the offspring of lesbian and gay parents will encounter hostility from peers during adolescence. Deevey (1989) has suggested that homophobia may in fact be especially intense among adolescents, who are in the process of developing their own sexual identity. Peer group prejudice and worry over possible stigmatization by friends appear to be major issues dealt with in therapeutic programs designed to address the concerns of adolescents in lesbian mother families. K. G. Lewis (1980) pointed to the sense of differentness and isolation felt by those children who know of no one else with a lesbian mother and therefore no one else with worries about friends' reactions if a mother's lesbian identity were to become known.

For children and adolescents, peer group stigmatization often manifests itself in the form of bullying. Bullying has been defined as an unprovoked and repeated physical or psychological hurt intentionally caused by either one child or a group of children to another child who generally feels powerless to retaliate (P. K. Smith, 1991). In the present study, young adults were asked if they had ever been teased or bullied by other pupils during their elementary, middle, or high school years. If they answered in the affirmative, they were asked to describe the most serious episode. When peer group stigmatization was reported, it was rated either as an "isolated incident" or as a "prolonged episode." All interviewees were also specifically asked to recall whether they had ever been teased or bullied about their own sexuality (either labeled as "gay/lesbian" or as a "sissy/tomboy") and whether they had ever been teased about their mother's lifestyle or about not having a father.

Table 5.3 displays the proportion of young adults in each group who reported having been teased or bullied during adolescence, with subjects categorized according to whether the incident was a minor isolated event or a more serious or prolonged episode over the course of an academic year. Young adults from lesbian mother families were no more likely to remember peer group hostility than were those from heterosexual single-parent homes. Furthermore, for those who reported peer group hostility, there was no group difference in the recollected seriousness of the episode. Being bullied by peers is not an uncommon ex-

TABLE 5.3. Experience of Peer Group Stigmatization by Family Type

		Lesbian mother	Heterosexual mother	Fisher's exact p
Peer group stigma	Peer teasing	20	15	NS
	No peer teasing	5	6	
Extent of peer stigma[a]	Prolonged episode	12	7	NS
	Isolated	8	8	
Peer stigma concerning own sexuality[a]	Peer teasing	11	4	.091
	No peer teasing	9	11	
Peer stigma concerning mother's lifestyle[a]	Peer teasing	9	3	NS
	No peer teasing	11	12	

Note. From Tasker and Golombok (1995). Copyright 1995 by the American Orthopsychiatric Association, Inc. Reprinted by permission.
[a]Those who reported no peer group stigmatization were excluded from these analyses.

perience for schoolchildren. In the present study, 76% (35/46) of all interviewees reported that they had been teased or bullied at some point during their school career, with 41% describing a prolonged or serious episode of intimidation by peers.

Here, as elsewhere in this book, it is appropriate to place the findings in the context of recent British data when these are available. From their survey of the prevalence of bullying among English schoolchildren, Whitney and Smith (1993) estimated that, on average, 27% of junior and middle school pupils are bullied sometimes, while 10% are bullied once a week or more. Ten percent of high school students in the same study reported that they had been bullied at least once during the preceding term, and 4% reported having been bullied once a week or more. The in-depth questioning on recollections of teasing and bullying over the entire school career probably accounts for the higher rates found in the present study.

In our study we found a nonsignificant trend suggesting that those from lesbian mother families were likely to recall having been teased about being gay or lesbian themselves (see Table 5.3). However, the groups did not differ with respect to the proportion of young adults who had been teased about their family background. For all subjects combined, those who had been teased about their family background were more likely to report having been teased about their own sexuality as well (Fisher's exact $p < .001$). For young women, no differences in reports of teasing, either about their own sexuality or about their mother's, were apparent between those from lesbian and those from heterosexual mother families, and there were no differences between those from middle-class lesbian and middle-class heterosexual mother families in this respect. However, of the six young men from lesbian mother families who mentioned teasing, four reported having been teased about their own sexuality, but only one of the nine young men from a heterosexual mother family remembered being teased in this way (Fisher's exact $p = .047$). The data from interviewees who came from working-class backgrounds revealed a nonsignificant trend suggesting that young people from lesbian mother families were more likely to report having been teased about their mother than were those from heterosexual mother families (4/7 vs. 2/15, respectively; Fisher's exact $p = .054$).

It seems, therefore, that children from working-class lesbian mother families may be more likely than those from middle-class lesbian mother families to experience peer stigma about issues connected with their mother's lesbian identity. In general, higher rates of bullying have been recorded in schools located in more socioeconomically disadvantaged areas (Whitney & Smith, 1993). And in a recent survey of British sexual attitudes and lifestyles, Wellings, Wadsworth, and Johnson (1994) reported that respondents with working-class backgrounds, and particularly those with lower educational qualifications, held less tolerant views of gay and lesbian relationships than did respondents with middle-class backgrounds.

Children from lesbian mother families may experience some aspects of "courtesy stigma," an expression coined to denote prejudice from being associated with a stigmatized group, a prejudice reported by other researchers of stigmatization (Goffman, 1963; Sigelman, Howell, Cornell, Cutright, & Dewey, 1991). Another explanation is that our interviewees from lesbian mother families were more sensitive to casual remarks from peers about sexual orientation and therefore remembered incidents that were more quickly forgotten by those in the comparison group. The following extract from Jeffrey's interview indicates his sensitivity to remarks made by peers and the significance he attached to being related to someone who identified herself as lesbian.

JEFFREY: I mean, people in school called me gay and queer and things at school. And I managed to say, "No I'm not" or "You are" or whatever, and then when I realized that my mum was, and it suddenly ＿＿＿ for a while I thought, "Maybe that's why they think I am or maybe that's why" ＿＿＿ and then it became clear that they didn't necessarily know that my mum was lesbian so while ＿＿＿ but I always avoided telling people. Very few friends of mine now or then knew. Very few.

Overall, the results of our research indicate that children in lesbian mother families are no more likely to experience teasing or bullying than are children from heterosexual single-parent or stepfamily backgrounds. However, in our study there was a tendency for young adults from lesbian mother families to report that peers had teased them about their own sexuality.

Who Are Teased about Family Background?

Recent legal rulings in custody cases have focused particularly on the likelihood of the child from a lesbian or gay family being stigmatized by peers ("B v B," 1991). It has been suggested that children with lesbian mothers who are politically active or are publicly "out" as lesbians in the local community may experience greater prejudice than those whose mothers maintain a low profile. Similarly, mothers and their children who spend much of their social life with lesbian women and gay men have been assumed to be more likely than those who do not experience prejudice. It has also been argued that children may be more likely to be exposed to teasing at school if their mother is insensitive to their possible need for secrecy and is not circumspect about letting her lesbian identity be known to her child's friends. The extent to which the family differs from the traditional heterosexual nuclear family stereotype has also been suggested as a factor influencing whether children are likely to experience peer group stigmatization. If the mother's female partner plays an active role in the child's life, this may attract unwanted attention to the family setup. Moreover, children who spend more time in their original traditional nuclear family before their mother identifies as lesbian may be less likely to experience peer stigma, as are those whose father continues to remain involved in their life.

Factors aside from immediate family circumstances may also influence whether children experience teasing. Other studies have found that victims of bullying are generally less popular with other children, and being able to call upon the loyalty of close friends may prevent teasing by the wider peer group (P. K. Smith, 1991). Therefore, children may be less likely to experience teasing if they have been able to form close friendships and if close friends are accepting of their family identity. The extent to which homosexuality is discussed and accepted within the local community is also likely to influence whether a child's peers at school are tolerant or hostile toward his or her lesbian mother family.

Because of the particular concern that children from lesbian mother families may encounter taunts about their own sexuality or about their mother, we examined whether different childhood experiences within the lesbian mother family group accounted for why some children from these families were teased while others were not. Tables 5.4 and 5.5 display point biserial correlations between variables from the initial and from the follow-up study, respectively, and young adults' reports of being teased during adolescence both about their lesbian mother and about their own sexual identity.

Table 5.5 shows that young adults whose father was supportive of their mother's lesbian relationship were less likely to report being teased about the mother's sexual identity by their peers ($r = -.619, p < .01$). Similarly, young adults who were not teased about their mother reported a closer relationship with their father at the time of follow-up ($r = -.502, p < .05$). This suggests that when fathers have a good relationship with the family, children brought up by lesbian mothers often avoid stigma, perhaps because they are less obviously families without male involvement. It is possible that peers are less likely to notice that a child's mother has a relationship with a woman if they know that the child's father is still around. However, there was no indication from the original study that a lack of contact between father and child is associated with peer group stigmatization. Therefore, it may not be the father's actual level of involvement but the child's perception of him as being supportive of the family that is the crucial issue. For example, Sonja talked about her relationship with her father and mother in the following way, emphasizing her father's involvement in her schooling and his respectability:

SONJA: [My father] used to come round a lot right up until the time I was about 13 to visit me every week, and [my mum and dad] would consult with each other about my career and what school and stuff and they seemed to get on okay. . . . I see them both as very separate people. There's stuff about my dad that I look up to as a parent, and there's things about my mum that I do, but in very different ways. . . . With my dad the fact that he's made quite a bit

TABLE 5.4. Correlations between Variables from the Initial Study and Young Adults' Reports of Peer Teasing about Mother's Lesbian Identity and Own Sexuality during Adolescence

	Teased about mother	Teased about own sexuality
Family relationships at time of initial study		
Mother's expressed warmth to child (0, "none"–5, "very warm")	.273 (24)	.196 (24)
Mother's relationship history (0, "four partners or fewer"–1, "more than four partners or concurrent relationships")	.359† (24)	.257 (24)
Quality of mother's relationship with her female partner (1, "fully harmonious"–5, "serious conflict")	−.787*** (13)	−.393 (13)
Mother and partner share child care (0, "mother and partner share"–1, "mother main caregiver")	−.141 (13)	−.225 (13)
Child's contact with father (0, "none"–2, "at least weekly")	−.284 (25)	−.058 (25)
Number of years child raised in heterosexual home	−.464* (24)	−.378† (24)
Mother's identity at time of initial study		
Mother's contentment with her sexual identity (1, "prefer to be heterosexual"–5, "positive about lesbian identity")	.343† (25)	.306 (25)
Mother's political involvement (0, "no involvement in lesbian/gay politics"–3, "frequent involvement")	.229 (25)	.095 (25)
Mother's involvement in lesbian groups (0, "no involvement"–2, "frequent attendance")	.216 (25)	−.114 (25)
Mother's openness about lesbian identity at time of initial study		
Mother "out" in local community (0, "no"–2, "public knowledge")	.272 (25)	−.005 (25)
Mother "out" to child's school teachers (0, "no"–2, "discussed with teachers")	.263 (25)	.006 (25)
Mother's attitude toward men (1, "negative"–5, "some sexual feelings toward men")	−.332 (25)	−.083 (25)
Peers' response at time of initial study		
Quality of child's peer relationships (0, "good"–2, "definite difficulties")	.141 (19)	.027 (19)

† $p < .10$; * $p < .05$; *** $p < .001$.

TABLE 5.5. Correlations between Variables Measured at Follow-Up
and Young Adults' Reports of Peer Teasing about Mother's Lesbian Identity
and Own Sexuality during Adolescence

	Teased about mother	Teased about own sexuality
Family relationships at follow-up		
Current relationship with mother (1, "very negative"–4, "very positive")	.020 (25)	–.003 (25)
Adolescent relationship with mother's partner (1, "very negative"–4, "very positive")	.149 (24)	.000 (24)
Current relationship with mother's partner (1, "very negative"–4, "very positive")	–.064 (24)	–.153 (24)
Mother's relationship style (1, "exclusive"–4, "nonexclusive")	.424* (24)	.379† (24)
Conflict in mother's primary relationship (1, "regular episodes of conflict"– 4, "no serious conflict")	.025 (22)	.097 (22)
Closeness of current relationship with father (1, "very negative"–4, "very positive")	–.502* (19)	–.142 (19)
Father's attitude toward mother's relation- ships (1, "opposed/upset"–3, "expressed support")	–.619** (17)	–.249 (17)
Mother's identity at follow-up		
Mother's contentment with her identity (1, "prefer to be heterosexual"–3, "very positive")	.205 (23)	.230 (23)
Mother's involvement in feminist politics (0, "not involved"–1, "feminist")	.022 (24)	.007 (24)
Mother's involvement in lesbian/gay rights politics (0, "not involved"–1, "involvement")	.233 (23)	.046 (23)
Mother's openness about lesbian identity and attitude toward child's friends at follow-up		
Mother's openess about her lifestyle in front of school friends (0, "discrete"–1, "too open")	.635** (23)	.481* (23)
Mother's response to school friends visiting home (1, "very unwelcoming"–3, "welcoming")	–.119 (25)	.162 (25)
Peers' response at follow-up		
Child's disclosure to friends (1, "friends didn't know"–4, "friends told")	.042 (23)	–.223 (23)
Child's friends' response (1, "very negative"–4, "positive")	–.418† (18)	–.418† (18)

† $p < .10$; * $p < .05$; ** $p < .01$.

of his life and done quite a lot of things and been quite successful, in a fairly traditional way. And he's quite—yeah, I think it's to do with the fact that he's got quite a nice house, really, and a good sense of humor and stuff.

Dan also talked about his mother and father both being involved in school matters:

F.T.: Nobody ever said anything to you at school about your mum and Sandie? [No.] Nobody knew about your mum being with Sandie at, say parents' evenings or anything?

DAN: No. I think that Mum and Dad would go to parents' evenings together. There's been a lot of contact between them once they'd split up. They were both interested in how I was getting on at school, and they would both go to parents' evenings.

Data from the original study showed that children who were older when their mother identified herself as lesbian (i.e., who had spent more time as part of a heterosexual family) were less likely to have been teased about their mother ($r = -.464$, $p < .05$) and also tended to be less likely to have been teased about their own sexuality ($r = -.378$, $p < .10$; see Table 5.4). This may be because they had spent more of their childhood with their father at home and therefore less time in a lesbian mother family. Alternatively, children who were older when their mother began a lesbian relationship may have been more able to avoid peer prejudice.

Few of the variables pertaining to the quality of their relationship with their mother or her partner were associated with young adults' reports of having been teased. However, young people whose mother reported a closer relationship with her partner at the time of the original study were more likely to report having been teased during adolescence about their mother being a lesbian ($r = -0.787$, $p < .001$; see Table 5.4). Couples with a good relationship may have been more open about their lesbian relationship, thereby increasing the likelihood that the child's peers would become aware of the family's background.

There was also a nonsignificant trend suggesting that interviewees whose mother had reported a greater number of relationships at the time of the original study were more likely to report having been teased during adolescence about their family ($r = .359, p < .10$; see Table 5.4). Data from the follow-up interviews also showed the mother's relationship style to be associated with the child's having been teased about his or her family ($r = .424, p < .05$) and with a tendency for the child to have been teased about his or her own sexuality ($r = .379, p < .10$; see Table 5.5). This further supports the suggestion, discussed in Chapter 4, that mothers who have a greater number of relationships appear more openly lesbian than do those who have a long-term relationship with a special partner. For example, in her interview Amy talked about her mother's relationship with her partner, Cindy, which ended when Cindy wanted to have an open-relationship. Amy thought the relationship between the women was initially a very happy one, but the open affection they showed for one another caused her to worry that her friends might see them.

AMY: They were very special to one another, and the more they gave to one another the closer they became. Then the more acceptable Cindy was to me. So Cindy was treating my mum really well. . . . Sometimes, if we were to say go out on a Sunday, Mum and Cindy would hold hands. I was always so frightened that somebody from school was going to see it.

As shown in Table 5.5, young adults' reports of their mother being more open in front of their school friends than they would have wished was associated with teasing by peers, both about their mother being a lesbian ($r = .635, p < .01$) and about their own sexual identity ($r = .481, p < .05$). It is likely, however, that children who had been teased would then have construed their mother's actions as indiscreet. Whether their mother was "out" about her lesbian identity in the local community or actively involved in lesbian politics was not associated with young adults' recollections of being teased, perhaps because these aspects of the mother's life went unnoticed by peers at school.

The support of others outside the home also tends to relate

to whether children from lesbian mother families are likely to encounter peer group teasing or hostility. In our study there were two nonsignificant trends suggesting that young adults whose close friends at school were negative about their family background were more likely to experience teasing from the wider peer group about their mother's identity ($r = -.418, p < .10$) and their own sexuality ($r = -.418, p < .10$; see Table 5.5). The interview material indicates that a close friend was sometimes able to mediate between the child and the wider peer group. The following excerpt from Anna's interview not only illustrates the intense hurt often felt by those children who experience bullying but also the social pressure applied to them to display a heterosexual relationship to quell the homophobic accusations made by peers:

ANNA: I got to about 13 and, um, one of my friends at school, she weren't talking to me about something, that were it. She used to sleep overnight [at my house], and she said, "Well, where does so-and-so sleep?" And I said, "Well, with my mum," and she says, "Well, they don't, do they?" And I said, "Yeah, you know, they sleep together." And she says, "Ooh no." And that friend has gone to school and said, "Oh, Anna's mum sleeps with another woman, you know." . . . I wasn't allowed to go to her house anymore; her mum and dad forbid me from going anywhere near. And that hurt me because she'd been my best friend for a long, long time. . . . And I lost that friend and then, of course, a chain reaction. Everybody found out: "If you go near her, she's only like her mum; she'll just turn out like her mum, so you don't want to be near her." . . . But there were one friend that really did stick by me, and she's still around.

F. T.: Would you say she was your closest friend?

ANNA: Yeah, yeah. . . . I suppose Caroline is, yeah. . . . All I can remember is Carline being there and everybody just coming round basically to what Caroline was saying to them, so that was that.

F. T.: Yes, right. So Caroline was actually quite important then?

ANNA: Yeah, because, as I say, she sort of were the one who said, "Look, she's not like you say; she, you know, she's a nice person," and what have you. But not long after that I met Hugh, . . . so, er, it tended to be sort of first boyfriend, totally addicted to him, never went anywhere without him, anyway. . . . It was just sort of that everybody was going through that stage, anyway, where they only wanted boyfriends and then they weren't really bothered, you know. As long as they were in the background, they left you.

F. T.: So when people at school started getting boyfriends, that actually meant they lost interest. Is that right?

ANNA: Well, it did me a favor, really, because once I started going out with Hugh, um, they looked at me different. They must have thought, "Well, she's not like we were saying she were because she's got a boyfriend, you know."

ATTITUDES TOWARD LESBIAN AND GAY RIGHTS AND WOMEN'S RIGHTS

Since young people's attitudes are highly correlated with their perceptions of their parents' attitudes (Acock & Bengston, 1980; Noller & Callan, 1991), recent writers have suggested that children from lesbian and gay families might be more able to appreciate cultural diversity and hold less conservative views on minority rights (Rafkin, 1990; Patterson, 1992). It has also been suggested that gay men and lesbian women who play an active and responsible role in the community may increase children's acceptance of homosexuality and nontraditional gender roles (Riddle, 1978).

In the present study, we examined whether young adults from lesbian mother families hold more liberal views on gay rights and women's rights than do their peers from heterosexual mother families. Young adults' attitudes toward gay and lesbian rights were rated on a 4-point scale: 1 (opposed to gay men or lesbian women), 2 (tolerant), 3 (positive, that is, previously spoken up for gay men or lesbian women) and 4 (active in the cause of gay or lesbian rights). Interviewees from both types of family background were asked specifically whether they felt that gay men or lesbian women are discriminated against in society, whether they had ever argued against prejudice directed at gay men or lesbian women, and whether they had been politically active in support of gay rights. The interviewee's general attitude toward gay men and lesbian women, as revealed during the course of the interview, was also taken into consideration in the final rating. In addition, all interviewees were asked whether their mother had been involved in feminist politics, and those from lesbian mother families were also asked whether their mother had been involved in lesbian or gay rights campaigns. A rating of general attitude toward lesbian women and gay men was made for the heterosexual mothers on the basis of their son's or daughter's report.

As predicted, young people from lesbian mother families expressed significantly more positive attitudes toward gay men and lesbian women than did young adults from heterosexual backgrounds ($t = 3.49$, $df = 42$, $p < .001$). This result remained significant when those who had had a gay or lesbian relationship themselves were excluded from the analysis.

For all interviewees combined, those who came from middle-class backgrounds expressed significantly more positive attitudes toward gay rights than did those from working-class backgrounds ($t = -3.73$, $df = 42$, $p < .001$). In comparison with the group of single heterosexual mothers, more of the lesbian mothers in our sample had received a college education and were rated as middle-class (see Chapter 3). Therefore, young adults from working-class and middle-class backgrounds were considered separately to establish whether those from lesbian homes were indeed more positive in their views, irrespective of social class. No group difference was found for those from working-class backgrounds. However, interviewees from middle-class lesbian mother families showed a trend although not statistically significant, toward greater support of lesbian and gay rights as compared to their counterparts from heterosexual middle-class families ($t = 1.87$, $df = 21$, $p < .10$). Social class, therefore, seems to influence attitudes toward lesbian and gay rights in the direction of more positive attitudes among the middle class. There was also some indication that among young people from middle-class families those with lesbian mothers tend to be more positive.

Aside from general attitudes toward gay men and lesbian women, we considered whether young adults with lesbian mothers are more likely than those with heterosexual mothers to report having a gay or lesbian friend in their own social circle. Interviewees from lesbian mother families were more likely to report this to be the case than were those from heterosexual mother families (16/21 vs. 8/21, respectively; Fisher's exact p = .014). Within the sample overall, there was a nonsignificant trend suggesting that women rather than men tended to be more likely to report a lesbian or gay friend (16/23 vs. 8/19, respectively; Fisher's exact p = .070). It is therefore possible that the higher proportion of women from lesbian mother families in the sample influenced the overall group difference. Indeed, when considering only women, those from heterosexual mother families were just as likely as those from lesbian mother families to report a gay or lesbian friend. However, our analysis revealed a trend in the data suggesting that young men from lesbian mother families tended to be more likely than men from heterosexual mother families to report having a gay or lesbian friend (5/7 vs. 3/12, respectively; Fisher's exact p = .067).

Since interviewees who expressed greater support for gay rights generally came from middle-class backgrounds, it was not surprising that those from middle-class homes tended to be more likely to report a previous or current friendship with someone identified as gay or lesbian (16/23 of respondents from middle-class homes as opposed to only 8/19 of those from working class homes; Fisher's exact p = .070). There was, however, no indication, for either working-class or middle-class participants, that interviewees from lesbian mother families were more likely to have a gay or lesbian friend than were their peers from heterosexual households. It seems that social class has a stronger effect on attitudes toward lesbian and gay rights and on friendship formation than does family background.

When coding attitudes toward women's rights, we divided interviewees according to whether they professed no interest (or antipathy) in women's rights or expressed a general awareness of and interest in women's rights (either by defining themselves as feminists or by championing women's rights when arguing with others). Those from lesbian mother families (12/22) were no more likely than those from heterosexual mother families (14/20) to express general support for women's rights.

Whether their mother sympathized with feminist issues did

not make any difference in the attitude toward women's rights of those brought up in heterosexual mother families. In contrast, young adults from lesbian mother families did express more support for women's rights if their mother sympathized with feminist causes (10/13), whereas none of the nine young adults whose lesbian mothers were not interested in feminist issues expressed support for women's rights (Fisher's exact; $p < .001$). Alan's mother was both a lesbian and a feminist, and he described how this had given him a different perspective on gender and on gay and lesbian issues:

ALAN: I think I've ended up looking at males from a feminist point of view. I haven't been conditioned by my mum at all, because I've always been given my own freedom of choice. But because I've been brought up by my mum in female relationships etcetera, I've sort of stepped back and looked at males from a slightly exterior point of view. And they really do look inferior, and they really do look the sort of more silly kind of species, compared to females that I know. 'Cause I mean in my opinion the females go through so much more than males and put up with it a lot more.

F. T.: Have you been involved in any student groups discussing, say, gender issues?

ALAN: No. You mean active groups? I've always remained my own opinion type person, and I'm not really going to put it on anyone else. I mean gays and lesbians have come up a hell of a lot in my life. That's the one big point I will argue for, you know, but otherwise not really.

F. T.: Have you been involved in any protests about gay rights or anything like that?

ALAN: I haven't been involved directly in protests. I mean, I agree with what the gays and lesbians are fighting for, but I haven't actually gone the step further to become active in that.

SUMMARY

In our study, children from lesbian mother families were no more likely than their counterparts from heterosexual single-parent families to experience peer stigma during adolescence, and most were able to integrate close friends with family life. When asked about their general experience of being teased or bullied, young adults from lesbian mother families were no more likely to report victimization than were those from heterosexual single-parent homes. Furthermore, they were no more likely to recollect being teased specifically about their mother. However, there was a nonsignificant trend suggesting that young people from lesbian mother families were more likely to recollect peer group teasing about their own sexuality. Within the lesbian mother family group, those who remembered being teased either about their own sexuality or about their mother's sexual identity were more likely to feel that their mother had been too open about lesbian issues in front of their friends. There is also evidence to suggest that children who felt that their father was not supportive of their mother's lesbian identity were more likely to remember being teased about their mother's identity.

The young adults from lesbian households in our study distinguished between concern over the possible reaction to their family of peers in general and concern over the more specific response of friends. Over half were able to selectively inform a close friend who did not react in a negative way or tell others. Although children's peer relationships were not necessarily adversely affected by being raised in a lesbian mother family, that is not to say that those who experienced bullying did not suffer. Furthermore, many young adults from lesbian mother families reported feeling some concern during adolescence that if other children found out about their family background, they might be hostile.

In general, we found that social class appears to have a stronger influence than family background on attitudes toward gay and lesbian rights, although there is some evidence to suggest that young adults from middle-class lesbian mother families are more likely to hold positive attitudes toward gay men and lesbian women than are those from middle-class heterosexual mother families. Our data show that young people from lesbian mother families are no more likely than their counterparts from heterosexual backgrounds to express support for women's rights, although it appears that young adults whose lesbian mothers hold feminist views are the ones who are most likely to champion equal opportunities for women.

CHAPTER SIX

Intimate Relationships

W HEN LESBIAN parenthood is debated in the legal or public arena, one of the most frequently raised issues is whether children's own intimate relationships will be influenced by being brought up in a lesbian mother family. In the first part of this chapter we consider whether young people raised by a lesbian mother are more likely to be attracted to and have relationships with partners of the same gender than are young people from heterosexual mother families. We also examine how much maternal support young adults with lesbian and heterosexual mothers receive in the formation of their early relationships and to what extent they communicate with their mother about sexual and relationship matters. Finally, findings relating to the overall patterns of the young adults' intimate relationships are discussed.

SEXUAL ORIENTATION

In the previous chapter we learned that other children often believe that children from lesbian mother households are more likely to be lesbian or gay themselves, probably reflecting a belief that is widespread in society. However, as discussed in Chapter 2, there is no evidence from the few studies that have so far been published on this topic that lesbian mothers are more likely to have gay sons or lesbian daughters (Patterson, 1992).

The various theoretical explanations of the development of sexual orientation reviewed in Chapter 2 provided the framework for examining whether children brought up by lesbian mothers are more likely than their counterparts from heterosexual backgrounds to develop a lesbian or gay sexual orientation. Traditional psychoanalytic theorists suggest that relinquishing their preoedipal libidinal attachment to their mother may be more problematic for both boys and girls if they are unable to develop a relationship with their father: "A boy or girl who has a good warm relationship with a heterosexual father does not become an overt homosexual" (Fine, 1987, p. 91). One of the leading proponents of the Kleinian object relations school, Hanna Segal, also has argued that the masculinity (and, by implication, the sexuality) of a boy brought up by a lesbian couple is less secure (Rose, 1990). Psychoanalytic theorists generally hold the view that children who fail to identify with their same-sex parent at the completion of the oedipal period are more likely to identify as gay or lesbian when they grow up. The quality of the child's relationships with the mother and father is considered to be an important determinant of the child's resolution of the oedipal dilemma. The combination of a domineering mother and a weak father is thought to lead to a homosexual orientation for boys whereas for girls a lesbian orientation is thought to originate in a hostile and fearful relationship with the mother.

Predictions derived from classical social learning theory claim that children model behaviors exhibited by their same-gender parent and that parental reinforcement for such behavior encourages children's imitations (Mischel, 1966, 1970; Bandura, 1977, 1986, 1989). However, whether or not an adult is imitated by a child seems to depend upon the child's a priori conception of the gender appropriateness of the model's behavior (Perry & Bussey, 1979; Huston, 1983). More recently, social learning theorists have emphasized the importance of peers, other adults, the mass media, and, in particular, the role of gender stereotypes in promoting conventional gender role behavior. It is thought that children learn about the behavior of both sexes through observation and that homosexual men and women are devalued in heterosexual society.

From the perspective of social learning theory it might be expected that lesbian mothers who are more open about same-gender relationships in front of their children, who wish their children to develop a lesbian or gay identity, or who reinforce their children's same-gender attractions would be more likely to have children who would themselves develop a lesbian or gay sexual orientation. Nevertheless, children raised in a lesbian household have been exposed to a predominantly heterosexist society outside the home; alternative models of heterosexual behavior and sources of reinforcement for heterosexual conduct are therefore widely available.

Symbolic interactionist and social constructionist theorists argue that sexual identity is constructed throughout the life course as the person becomes aware of different cultural scenarios for socially appropriate sexual encounters and develops both internal fantasies associated with sexual arousal and interpersonal scripts for sexual relationships with others (Simon & Gagnon, 1987; Gagnon, 1990). Plummer (1975) proposed that childhood experiences, such as genital play with someone of the same gender and same-gender emotional attachments and fantasies, create a potential source for "homosexual identification." Other phenomena—such as having a particular body build, displaying cross-gendered behavior, and experiencing feelings of being separate or different from peers—may also lead to homosexual identification because of cultural associations between these phenomena and later homosexuality. Plummer suggests that many people have same-gender sexual experiences at some point in their life although few develop a homosexual identity. From an interactionist perspective an important part is played by identification with significant others, who enable an individual to either neutralize a homosexual potential or construct a gay or lesbian identity. For example, a lesbian mother family context may provide the child with an immediate reference group, thus enabling the child to readily label same-gender experiences and feelings as homosexual. Furthermore, through the family the young person may already have socialized with other lesbian women and with gay men and may be aware of different lesbian and gay cultures. Therefore, the process of "coming out" and identifying as gay or lesbian may be facilitated.

Women's involvement in different types of heterosexual and lesbian partnerships is of central concern to feminists, who argue for equality and women's empowerment in relationships (see Cartledge & Ryan, 1983). Intimate relationships are seen not just as reflections of personal preference but also as created by and in response to heteropatriarchal society, where the dominant social expectations lead to the assumption of a heterosexual identity. It is argued that unless they have access to different discourses, most young people are given no choice but to become heterosexual. However, the situation may be different for children brought up in lesbian mother families, particularly if their mother holds a feminist political perspective. Feminist mothers in the present study were defined on the basis of sons' and daughters' reports of their mother's involvement in women's rights campaigns. This included mothers who probably would have described themselves as radical feminists as well as others for whom the rejection of men as sexual partners was not central to their feminist analysis. It is reasonable to suppose that while they were growing up, daughters of feminist mothers may well have heard discussions about relationship alternatives for empowering women, discussions that may have led them to question the automatic assumption of a heterosexual identity, to become more aware of same-gender feelings, and to consider choosing a lesbian lifestyle for themselves.

In the follow-up interviews, data on sexual orientation were gathered through questioning about friendships, crushes, and sexual fantasies, experiences, relationships, and identity during adolescence and adulthood. Data on psychosexual behavior were always collected toward the end of the interview, by which time rapport had generally been established. This section of the interview commenced with questions on experience of prepubertal sexual play with same-gender and opposite-gender children. Interviewees were then asked about their interest in other children's bodies and physical development during puberty. As well as soliciting information, these background questions encouraged interviewees to consider sexual curiosity about others in a nonthreatening way prior to being asked about their sexual attractions and relationships during adolescence and adulthood. The young men and women were then asked to recall their first and subsequent crushes from the beginning of puberty to their first sexual relationship in order to establish the extent of same-gender and opposite-gender attraction in their lives. They were asked if they had ever been physically attracted to a friend and if they had ever had sexual fantasies about someone of the same gender.

Interviewees were also asked if they had ever previously thought during adolescence that they might become involved in lesbian or gay relationships and if they currently thought it possible that they might have lesbian or gay relationships in the future. A chronological sexual relationship history was then obtained from each interviewee; this described all of the sexual relationships the person had experienced with each relationship being assessed in terms of the person's age when the relationship began, the partner's gender, the level of sexual intimacy in the relationship, the length of the relationship, and whether marriage or cohabitation with the partner had occurred (and, if so, the length of the relationship prior to marriage or cohabitation).

It has been recommended by Richardson (1983) that sexual orientation be conceptualized along three separate dimensions: desire for someone of the same gender, sexual contact with a partner of the same gender, and identification as lesbian, gay, or bisexual. To ascertain whether growing up in a lesbian household influences sexual orientation, we analyzed the interview data according to these dimensions (see also Golombok & Tasker, 1996). Moreover, since consideration of the possibility of having a lesbian or gay relationship is distinct from the experience of same-gender desire, this aspect of sexual orientation was also examined.

Same-Gender Sexual Attraction

Interviewees were divided according to whether they reported any same-gender physical attraction as opposed to only opposite-gender attraction. Sexual attraction was defined in terms of the object of crushes and fantasies; this is equivalent to categorizing participants on a Kinsey scale with a rating of 1 and above for fantasy (Kinsey, Pomeroy, & Martin, 1948, 1953; Sandfort, van Zessen, & de Vroome, 1994). As shown in Table 6.1, children brought up in lesbian households were no more likely than their peers from heterosexual households to be attracted to someone of the same gender. Nine children of lesbian mothers (six daughters and three sons) and four children of heterosexual mothers (two daughters and two sons) reported same-gender attraction. When the analysis was repeated for men and women separately, no differences were found between the two family types.

TABLE 6.1. Young Adults' Experience of Same-Gender Attraction and Consideration of Lesbian/Gay Relationships and Sexual Identity by Family Type

		Lesbian mother	Heterosexual mother[a]	Fisher's exact p
Same-gender sexual attraction	Same-gender attraction	9	4	
	Opposite-gender attraction only	16	16	NS
Consideration of lesbian/gay relationships	Future possibility	6	2	
	Previously considered	8	1	
	Never considered	8	15	.003[b]
Same-gender sexual relationship	Same-gender relationship	6	0	
	No same-gender relationship	19	20	.022
Sexual identity	Bisexual/lesbian/gay identity	2	0	
	Heterosexual identity	23	20	NS

Note. Adapted from Golombok and Tasker (1996). Copyright 1996 by the American Psychological Association. Reprinted by permission.
[a]Data on sexual orientation were unavailable for one male participant.
[b]Fisher's exact test *p* calculated for previous/future consideration of lesbian/gay relationships versus never considered gay/lesbian relationships.

Consideration of Same-Gender Relationships

Closer examination of the interview material suggested that young adults from lesbian mother families held attitudes that were different from those of their counterparts from heterosexual mother families toward being attracted to someone of the same gender. In general, those from heterosexual homes had never considered that there were alternatives to heterosexuality. When they did sometimes report a strong emotional attachment to someone of the same gender, these feelings were thought of as a "special friendship" and no attraction was acknowledged. For example:

F. T.: What about feelings of attraction or romantic feelings to any boys that you knew?

AARON: No, I've never had any of that.

F. T.: Or feeling of a special relationship?

AARON: I think me and Kevin have got a special relationship, because I just trust him implicitly, I suppose. Um, I suppose everything I've done, you know, we've done together sort of thing. We hitched across Europe, er, in the summer holidays when I was 14. So we've done quite a lot of things together and we've known quite a lot of people and we've always stuck together. Even though like there might have been a lot of mates, it's quite clear that we stick together.

F. T.: Yeah, you're best mates sort of thing. [Yeah.] Have you ever felt attracted to him or not?

AARON: No, no not really.

F. T.: Like you want to touch him or anything like that?

AARON: I've put my arm round him. Um, on occasions we've even given each other a kiss goodbye sort of thing, but I don't ____ I've never seen it as a sexual thing. It's like we're that close that we can do that.

F. T.: When you say you've given him a kiss good-bye, when does that happen?

AARON: It's usually when we've had a drink (laughs). Sort of, er, well, over the last—um, what? year or two—we don't see, er, that much of each other now, because I live with my girlfriend and he lives down the other end of London. Well, no, that's irrelevant really (laughs). Actually, er, well, on occasions when I've given him a kiss or he's given me a kiss, it's like, er, I don't know ____ it didn't, um ____ I think it was done more of in a macho sort of way, really. It might be hard to understand.

F. T.: Have you ever had any sexual fantasies or erotic dreams or anything about men or gay dreams or whatever. Do you ever remember anything like that?

AARON: No.

F. T.: Have you ever thought about gay relationships for yourself or thought about experimenting with other men?

AARON: Um, no, I've never really wondered what it was like at all.

In contrast, young adults who had been brought up in lesbian households and who identified as heterosexual had often thought about whether their mother's sexual orientation had any implications for their own sexual identity. They were more likely to recognize that interactions with same-gender friends had possibilities for the development of intimate relationships. However, this did not mean that they necessarily felt physically attracted to others of the same gender, or that they were contemplating a gay or lesbian relationship. For example, Lois's response to questioning about same-gender attraction reflected an awareness of permeable boundaries between friendship and attraction:

F. T.: What about any fantasies about girls or women?

LOIS: No, never. I'm afraid not. I have to disappoint you there (*laughs*). No, I didn't. No, never.

F. T.: And any physical experience with women?

LOIS: No.

F. T.: What about with friends? Has there ever been any sort of romantic involvement there?

LOIS: What, with girlfriends? No. I mean, I went through the sort of stage of thinking that I was lesbian because of the mere fact that I realized suddenly that I loved my friends, you know, and I wanted to hug them good-bye and things. And so I think probably because I knew my mother was gay, I was a lot more cautious about things like that, you know, 'cause I wouldn't _____ 'cause it would be, "Oh, my God, I'm gay, I'm gay," so I used to steer clear totally. Not that I ever came into contact, anyhow.

For those children from lesbian mother families who had examined their own sexual and emotional feelings in this context, an awareness of the choice between same- and opposite-gender partners was able to produce temporary feelings of uncertainty, as in Lois's case. However, it was also able to open possibilities for sexual exploration or for the development of a new sexual identity:

BARBARA: I must admit I would like to go to bed with Wilma, 'cause sexual pleasure I get I would know how. I know where my erogenous zones are, where I like to be touched and stroked, and to be able to do that instinctively with somebody, with another woman, because a fella's erogenous zones are in a different place (*laughs*). I would very much like to go to bed with Wilma, but I don't think that makes me a lesbian or a homosexual or anything.

F. T.: Have you thought about taking it further?

BARBARA: Yes, possibly. They say, "Don't knock it until you've tried it," don't they? . . . I wouldn't mind trying, but I don't know. Like I say, I wouldn't want to go to bed with anyone else; I'd only want to go to bed with Wilma.

F. T.: So for you it would just be experimenting?

BARBARA: Yes.

F. T.: And not necessarily moving into a lesbian relationship?

BARBARA: Yeah, it would purely be just experimentation, and I would very much like to, but I don't think I would enjoy . . . but I don't think I would want to become a full-time lesbian.

F. T.: Why not?

BARBARA: Er, um, I just don't think I'd enjoy sex with a woman as much as I do with a man.

The interviewees were categorized according to whether they had never thought of the possibility of same-gender relationships for themselves, whether they had previously thought that they might experience same-gender attraction or relationships, or whether they thought it possible that they might do so in the future. Significantly more of the young adults from lesbian than from heterosexual mother families stated that they had previously considered that they might experience same-gender sexual attraction or have a same-gender sexual relationship or stated that they considered such experiences possible in the future (Fisher's exact $p = .003$; see Table 6.1). Fourteen children of lesbian mothers (four sons and ten daughters) reported this to be the case, compared with three children of heterosexual mothers (two sons and one daughter). Daughters of lesbian mothers were significantly more likely than daughters of heterosexual mothers to consider that they might experience same-gender sexual attraction or have a lesbian relationship (Fisher's exact $p = .019$). There was no significant difference between sons from lesbian and heterosexual mother families for this variable.

In general, alternatives to a heterosexual identity were not considered or were dismissed as an option for themselves by interviewees from heterosexual family backgrounds—even when heterosexual relationships were not felt to be satisfying. For example, Deonne's thoughts on having another relationship with a man were as follows:

DEONNE: It's not something that I want to do, but, um, I think, "Well what else is there?" Being a spinster (*laughs*). Um, I really ____ I don't know. I feel quite negative about relationships at the moment and think "Oh well, no, I can't really," thinking "Oh no, I can't be bothered" and "They're not worth the bother." You know, stuff like that. But I don't know.

F. T.: Why, specifically, do you feel negative about relationships with men?

DEONNE: It's not just what happened to my mum and what she says. It's everybody (*laughs*), you know. I know so many people who, you know, um, in my sort of age group who are getting into relationships and they are not working that there doesn't seem like a lot of hope.

Same-Gender Sexual Relationships

Table 6.1 shows that significantly more young people from lesbian mother families than from heterosexual mother families reported having experienced a sexual relationship with someone of the same gender (Fisher's exact $p = .022$). None of the interviewees from heterosexual mother families reported a same-gender sexual relationship. In contrast, six young people (one son and five daughters) from lesbian mother families reported one or more relationships with a partner of the same gender. When this analysis was repeated for daughters only, a nonsignificant trend remained (Fisher's exact $p = .094$). These relationships varied from a brief encounter involving only kissing to lengthy cohabitation. In all cases, the interviewee experienced physical attraction to the same-gender partner. At the time of her follow-up interview Shona (age 20) had been with her current boyfriend for 5 months. During the interview she described her only sexual relationship with another woman (Tina), which ended 2 years prior to the interview.

SHONA: With Tina I was really worried because here I was with a woman and I really fancied her and I thought she really fancied me, but, like, if I didn't do something, nothing would have been done. But, um, I went over to visit her and we were being friendly towards each other and she just sort of made a pass at me and I ended up staying over.

Sexual Identity

The two groups of participants did not differ significantly with respect to sexual identity. All of the young adults with a heterosexual mother and the large majority of those with a lesbian mother identified themselves as heterosexual. Only two young women from lesbian mother families identified themselves as lesbian. Both were in a lesbian relationship at the time of follow-up and expressed a commitment toward lesbian relationships in the future. These women felt that having a lesbian mother had helped them to come out as lesbian but that their family background had not pushed them in this direction. It should also be noted that both women had previously experimented with heterosexual relationships.

F. T.: Do you feel that your family background, having a lesbian mother, has had any influence on your relationships?

MICHELLE: Well, not really, because ____ well, I don't know. I mean, I suppose ____ um, well, the obvious thing ____ I mean, when people find out that I've got a lesbian mother, then everyone sort of thinks, "Oh, that's why you're one then." But, you know I first started going out with blokes. I mean, so (sighs) ____ so I don't really think it's had that much effect.

F. T.: Do you think you'd have had lesbian relationships anyway?

MICHELLE: Well, I don't really know.

F. T.: Or that it's made it easier for you to have lesbian relationships?

MICHELLE: Yeah. I think it's made it easier for me to have, yeah, lesbian relationships. Because other friends have had horrendous times telling their parents. So, yeah, it's been really easy for me (*sighs*). I haven't had problems like that.

F. T.: But you don't feel it's had any other influence apart from that?

MICHELLE: I mean, in a way that it's tied in with the women's issues and things because I've been aware of that since I was a kid, although I might not have understood it particularly well or, you know, really been into it, but I have been aware of it. Like I say, this thing about Mum saying, "All men are the same" and me and [my sister] sort of saying, "No, you can't say that, can you, Mother?" You know, when we were younger and then getting back together later and we discussed it about a year ago or something and said, "She was right, wasn't she?"; "Yes, she was"; and that sort of thing. So, I mean, it's been ____ I've been more involved. Well, I know more about women's issues from an earlier age than I think a lot of people have. And, I mean, there's been parents obviously who've made it, um, very easy for me to accept that I can have feelings like that and not hide them forever.

At the time of follow-up, nine of the children from lesbian backgrounds (six daughters and three sons) had experienced same-gender attraction, fewer reported having same-gender relationships (five daughters and one son), and only two (both daughters) identified themselves as homosexual. Although estimates of the percentage of the general population who identify themselves as lesbian or gay or who have engaged in same-gender sexual relationships vary widely, the prevalence of homosexuality in the United States is currently thought to range from 4% to 17% (Gonsiorek & Weinrich, 1991). Thus, the finding that 2 of the 25 young adults raised by lesbian mothers identified themselves as lesbian does not appear to be inconsistent with general population norms, although the larger proportion of such young adults who had experienced a same-gender sexual relationship seems to be higher than would be expected in the general population. Estimates for the United Kingdom are somewhat lower, particularly for women. In the British National Survey of Sexual Attitudes and Lifestyles (Wellings et al., 1994), 6.1% of men and 3.4% of women reported some homosexual experience, and only 1.1% of men and 0.4% of women reported a gay or lesbian relationship in the preceding year. Furthermore, in a review of studies evaluating the rates of homosexuality and bisexuality in different countries, it was estimated that between 5% and 6% of males and between 2% and 3% of females had been involved in same-gender sexual relationships (Diamond, 1993).

Although our findings suggest that daughters of lesbian mothers may be more open than sons to same-gender sexual relationships, in the original study there was a higher ratio of daughters to sons in the lesbian mother group and a higher ratio of sons to daughters in the heterosexual group, which remained at follow-up. Thus, the higher proportion of women than men who reported consideration of and involvement in same-gender sexual relationships may reflect this sampling bias.

Factors Associated with Same-Gender Sexual Interest

Information on family background from both the original and the follow-up study was used to examine the family characteristics of young adults who expressed interest in same-gender sexual relationships. These findings are presented separately for the two groups of participants. From the data on same-gender attraction and relationships, a rating of same-gender sexual interest was made for each interviewee ranging from 0 (no same-gender attraction or same-gender sexual relationships), through 1 (same-gender attraction but no same-gender sexual relationships), to 2 (same-gender sexual attraction and same-gender sexual relationships).

It can be seen from Table 6.2 that for young adults from lesbian backgrounds several variables from the original study were correlated with same-gender sexual interest at follow-up. These

TABLE 6.2. Pearson Product–Moment Correlations between Childhood Family Characteristics and Young Adults' Same-Gender Sexual Interest

	Same-gender sexual interest	
	Lesbian mother	Heterosexual mother
Family relationships at the time of initial study		
Mother's expressed warmth to child (0, "none"–5, "very warm")	.094 (24)	.252 (19)
Mother's relationship history (0, "four partners or fewer"–1, "more than four partners or concurrent relationships")	.596** (25)	—
Quality of mother's relationship with her female partner (1, "fully harmonious"–5, "serious conflict")	.000 (13)	—
Mother and partner share child care (0, "mother and partner share"–1, "mother main caregiver")	.023 (13)	—
Child's contact with father (0, "none"–2, "at least weekly")	.280 (25)	.373 (20)
Number of years child raised in heterosexual home	.092 (25)	—
Mother's identity at time of initial study		
Mother's contentment with her sexual identity (1, "prefer to be heterosexual"–5, "positive about lesbian identity")	−.149 (25)	—
Mother's political involvement (0, "no involvement"–3, "frequent involvement")	.093 (25)	—
Mother's openness about lesbian identity at time of initial study		
Mother's openness in showing affection in front of child (0, "none"–2, "kiss/caress")	.735*** (18)	—
Mother's preference for child's sexual orientation (0, "prefer heterosexual"–1, "no preference")	.384† (25)	—
Mother "out" in local community (0, "no"–2, "public knowledge")	−.041 (25)	—
Mother "out" to child's school teachers (0, "no"–2, "discussed with schoolteachers")	.220 (25)	—
Mother's attitude toward men (1, "negative"–5, "some sexual feelings")	−.030 (25)	—

(*continued*)

TABLE 6.2. cont.

	Same-gender sexual interest	
	Lesbian mother	Heterosexual mother
Peers' response at time of initial study		
Quality of child's peer relationships	.189	.170
(0, "good"–2, "definite difficulties")	(19)	(14)
Child's characteristics at time of initial study		
Child's gender role behavior	.209	–.197
("gender typical"–"gender atypical")	(17)	(14)

Note. Adapted from Golombok and Tasker (1996). Copyright 1996 by the American Psychological Association. Adapted with permission.
† p < .10; ** p < .01; *** p < .001.

prospective findings are of particular interest because informa-tion about childhood family environment was obtained before the participants began to engage in sexual relationships; thus, the findings are not confounded by knowledge of their sexual orientation in adult life.[1]

Two variables from the original study were significantly cor-related with reports of same-gender sexual interest among young adults from lesbian mother families: Those who had a mother who was open to them about physical intimacy when they were school age ($r = .735, p < .001$) and those whose mother reported a greater number of lesbian relationships when they were school age ($r = .596, p < .01$) were more likely to report same-gender sexual interest. The following extract from Petra's interview il-lustrates the atmosphere of acceptance and openness about same-gender relationships in which she grew up:

PETRA: I remember the women's commune in a big sort of house we used to go to a lot. And there were like men kissing each other and women kissing each other and kids kissing each other, everyone used to kiss each other all the time, and I thought it was really nice, you know.

[1]Of the 25 young adults raised by lesbian mothers, 21 had not reached puberty when their family took part in the initial study. The correlations shown in Table 6.2 were all replicated excluding the four children who were older at the time of the original study.

None of the lesbian mothers in the original study expressed a wish for their children to be gay or lesbian when they grew up; neither did they encourage their children to develop same-gender attractions. However, there was a nonsignificant trend in the data suggesting that mothers who reported in the original study that they would accept their child's developing a non-heterosexual orientation tended to have children who at follow-up were more likely to report same-gender sexual interest ($r = .384$, $p < .10$; see Table 6.2). These mothers were also more likely to have had a greater number of relationships and were more open about physical intimacy in front of their children. When Holly reflected on whether her mother had ever expressed any preference for Holly's sexual orientation, the mother's acceptance of her daughter's relationship with another woman may have made it easier for Holly to express her feelings for Vivienne:

HOLLY: I don't think there was much [my mother] felt she could do to influence [my sexual orientation]. But she seemed to be really pleased when I was with Vivienne. . . . I think she was happier about me being with Vivienne than she's ever been about me being with a bloke.

In addition, young adults from lesbian mother families who reported at follow-up that their mother was involved in feminist politics were more likely to report same-gender sexual interest themselves ($r = .573$, $p < .01$; see Table 6.3). Mothers who were feminists also appeared to have been more open with their children about their sexual relationships, which may reflect an emphasis in the household on discussing of sexual relationships within the women's movement. It is important to remember, however, that the link between a mother's involvement in feminist politics and a child's later same-gender sexual interest may only be suggested by this cross-sectional data; no equivalent measure of the mother's involvement in feminist politics was available from the original study. No associations were identified between young adults' reports of same-gender sexual interest and measures of the mother's involvement in the gay rights movement as reported by mothers in the original study or as reported by sons and daughters at follow-up.

Only two variables measured at follow-up were associated with same-gender sexual interest among the young adults raised by heterosexual mothers (see Table 6.3). There was a nonsignificant trend suggesting that those who thought their mother was dissatisfied with her main relationship tended to be more likely to report same-gender sexual interest ($r = -.447$, $p < .10$), perhaps because seeing their mother experience an unhappy heterosexual relationship lead them to reflect on alternatives for themselves. There was also a nonsignificant trend ($r = .473$, $p < .10$) suggesting that young adults from heterosexual mother families who reported same-gender sexual interest also tended to be those who recollected playing sexual games during childhood with a same-gender peer (e.g., kissing and holding hands, viewing each other naked, and touching genitals). This supports Plummer's (1975) observation that childhood erotic or romantic experiences with same-gender friends may lead to recognition of homosexual feelings later in life. However, it is also plausible that interviewees who were aware of same-gender attractions had thought more about sexual play with friends in childhood or were more willing to admit to this during the interview.

For young adults from lesbian mother families, the variables that were found to be significantly associated with same-gender sexual interest all reflected their mother's openness with them about her own sexual identity, lending some support to a social cognitive theory explanation of children's development of sexual orientation. Children were more likely to report same-gender sexual interest if during childhood their mother had been accepting of the possibility of their adopting a nonheterosexual orientation. Possibly they were less likely than heterosexual mothers to reinforce their children for forming relationships with opposite-gender peers or, at least, were less likely to discourage them from same-sex relationships even if they did not actively encourage them. In addition, children were more likely to report same-gender sexual interest if their mother had been involved in several lesbian relationships and was more open about physical intimacy, thus providing a clearer model of lesbian relationships. These findings are also congruent with social constructionist and feminist explanations of sexual identity formation, which assume that seeing a variety of sexual scripts enables young people to

TABLE 6.3. Pearson Product–Moment Correlations between Characteristics at Follow-Up and Young Adults' Same-Gender Sexual Interest

	Same-gender sexual interest	
	Lesbian mother	Heterosexual mother
Family relationships at follow-up		
Current relationship with mother (1, "very negative"–4, "very positive")	− .214 (25)	.220 (20)
Adolescent relationship with mother's partner (1, "very negative"–4, "very positive")	− .337 (24)	.088 (19)
Current relationship with mother's partner (1, "very negative"–4, "very positive")	− .311 (24)	− .041 (17)
Mother's relationship style (1, "exclusive"–4, "nonexclusive")	.228 (24)	− .377 (19)
Mother's satisfaction with primary relationship (1, "very unhappy"–4, "very happy")	− .281 (23)	− .447† (23)
Conflict in mother's primary relationship (1, "regular episodes of conflict"– 4, "no serious conflict")	− .354 (22)	− .137 (22)
Closeness of current relationship with father (1, "very negative"–4, "very positive")	.149 (19)	.178 (12)
Father's attitude towards mother's relationships (1, "opposed/upset"–3, "expressed support")	.246 (17)	− .034 (10)
Mother's identity at follow-up		
Mother's contentment with her identity (1, "prefer to be heterosexual"–3, "very positive")	.010 (23)	− .268 (20)
Mother's involvement in feminist politics (0, "not involved"–1, "feminist")	.573** (24)	− .286 (18)
Mother's involvement in lesbian/gay rights politics (0, "not involved"–1, "involved")	.219 (23)	—
Mother's openness about lesbian identity and **attitude toward child's friends at follow-up**		
Mother's openness in showing physical affection in front of child (0, "interviewee not embarrassed" –1, "some embarrassment felt")	.027 (19)	.303 (16)
Extent to which adolescent talked to mother about sexual relationships (0, "never discussed"– 2, "ongoing discussion")	.246 (21)	− .054 (17)
Mother's attitude toward men (0, "negative"–1, "neutral or positive")	.201 (21)	− .033 (18)

(*continued*)

TABLE 6.3. *cont.*

| | Same-gender sexual interest | |
	Lesbian mother	Heterosexual mother
Peers' response at follow-up		
Teased about own sexuality	.228	.375
(0, "not teased"–1, "teased about sexuality")	(25)	(20)
Childhood experiences reported at follow-up		
Prepubertal sexual play with opposite-sex	−.339	.327
peers (0, "none"–1, "play experienced")	(24)	(20)
Prepubertal sexual play with same-sex	.138	.473†
(0, "none"–1, "play experienced")	(24)	(18)

† *p* < .10; ** *p* < .01.

consider same-gender sexual relationships for themselves. Their mother's openness about sexual identity and relationships may have enabled the sons and daughters of lesbian mothers to feel freer to explore and acknowledge their own sexual feelings.

The data from the present study give little support for psychoanalytic explanations of the origin of homosexual orientation, although our interviews may not have picked up on more subtle themes. None of the parent–child variables from the original investigation and none of the retrospective variables from the follow-up study, was significantly associated with young adults' reports of same-gender sexual interest. In addition, no association was identified between childhood gender role behavior at the time of the initial study and a young adult's report of same-gender sexual interest at follow-up, probably because the childhood gender role behavior of interviewees from both lesbian and heterosexual mother family backgrounds was typical for boys and girls of their age.

MOTHER–ADOLESCENT COMMUNICATION ABOUT SEXUAL RELATIONSHIPS

Surveys on adolescent sex education report that parents generally find it very difficult to talk to their sons and daughters about sexual relationships (Meikle, Peitchinis, & Pearce, 1985; Allen,

1987), and in custody disputes involving a lesbian mother it is often suggested that the heterosexual development of children brought up by lesbian mothers will be impeded by their mother's inability to discuss heterosexual relationships with them (Javaid, 1983). On the other hand, Riddle (1978) argued that adolescents may benefit from the increased self-acceptance of their own sexual identity that results from social interaction with gay men and lesbian women who can provide positive role models for interpersonal relationships.

In the follow-up interviews, young adults were asked about the extent to which they had been able to talk to their mother (or her partner) about problems in their own relationships; in particular, they were asked whether they had been able to discuss with their family their own sexual feelings and contraceptive needs during adolescence. They were also asked how welcoming or disapproving their mother or her partner had been of their own partners, if their mother had allowed them to have a partner sleep over with them while they were still living at home, and if they thought their mother had any preference regarding their sexual orientation.

The results displayed in Table 6.4 show that young people from lesbian mother families generally felt more able to discuss their own sexual development with their mother or her partner than did children brought up by single heterosexual mothers ($t = 3.64$, $df = 36$, $p < 0.01$), and there was no indication that daughters found it easier than sons to communicate with lesbian mothers about sexual matters. Five girls (two from heterosexual mother families and three from lesbian mother families) who had conflictual relationships with their mother were not included in these analyses, because they had told their mother about their sexual relationships during an argument rather than in the context of supportive sex education. Generally, the interviews with young people indicated not only that lesbian mothers were more able to offer advice on contraception but also that they were more aware of how sexually experienced their son or daughter was and were therefore able to discuss sexual issues as they arose. This was so irrespective of whether the adolescent had lesbian, gay, or heterosexual relationships. Here, for example, is Phillip's discussion of his mother's attitude toward his first experience of heterosexual intercourse.

TABLE 6.4. Young Adults' Communication with Their Mother about Sex Education by Family Type

	Lesbian mother		Heterosexual mother[a]	
	Male	Female	Male	Female
No communication	1	4	8	4
General communication about contraception	3	7	2	3
Discussed first sexual relationship	3	3	0	0

[a]Young adults from lesbian mother families versus young adults from heterosexual mother families ($t = 3.64$, $df = 36$, $p < .01$).

PHILLIP: It was like a one-night stand. I wanted it to be serious but I just met this girl at a party and before I knew it we were kissing and all of a sudden she said, "Do you want to spend the night with me?" And I was really shocked and I went out and I asked my mum. She said do whatever feels best. It was like a momentous occasion, and we ended up sleeping the night together.

F. T.: At your mum's?

PHILLIP: No, at a friend of my mum's. Um, very, very aware male, you know. I took precautions and all that.

The results of a study of sex education in the United Kingdom (Allen, 1987) revealed that in the mid-1980s only around 15% of boys and 35% of girls in a sample of 14- to 16-year-olds reported having discussed contraception with their mother. Parental embarrassment was the main reason given by both children and parents as to why so few parents had been able to discuss this issue. The finding in the present study that lesbian mothers are often better able than heterosexual mothers to talk to adolescents about contraception suggests that in deciding to be open about their lesbian relationships within the family circle, lesbian mothers are less embarrassed about discussing other sexual issues with their children.

However, the conversations that young people recalled with their mother indicated that mothers rarely went into detail about sexual relationships. If the young person was not interested in gay or lesbian relationships themselves, then most mothers, like Natalie's, did not discuss intimacy:

F. T.: Did you ever discuss with your mum the possibility of you having gay relationships?

NATALIE: Well, you mean like "Mum, what would you say if I said I was gay?" Well I would have thought, you know, that it was a foregone conclusion that if I was gay, she wouldn't really say anything. No, she wouldn't really say it was horrible or anything. No, I never mention it, but I don't think she would ever raise it. . . .

F. T.: The issue never really came up about gay relationships?

NATALIE: No, it wasn't something that I felt I wanted, so there wasn't really a lot of point in discussing it or thinking about it really 'cause it wasn't something that appealed to me.

Lesbian mothers were no more liberal than heterosexual mothers in allowing their adolescent son or daughter to have a partner sleep overnight with them in the home, even though they appeared to be more understanding of their adolescent son's or daughter's sexual development. Excluding those young people who were not sexually active while living at home, 8 of 18 adolescents from lesbian backgrounds and 8 of 17 adolescents from heterosexual households were allowed to have partners stay overnight in their room with their mother's consent.

The young people who participated in the follow-up study were asked whether they thought that their mother preferred them to be homosexual or heterosexual or whether they thought she had no preference regarding their sexual orientation. Not surprisingly, the results displayed in Table 6.5 show that young people from lesbian mother families were far more likely than those from heterosexual homes to think that their mother preferred them to be homosexual (Fisher's exact $p < .0001$). This finding reflects a difference between lesbian and heterosexual mothers' views regarding daughters (Fisher's exact $p = .006$) rather than sons. In only two of the ten cases in which interviewees thought their mother preferred them to be homosexual was this an issue

TABLE 6.5. Young Adults' Perceptions of Their Mother's Preference Regarding Their Sexual Orientation by Family Type

	Lesbian mother		Heterosexual mother		Fisher's exact p^a
	Male	Female	Male	Female[b]	
Prefer child to be heterosexual	4	4	6	7	$p < .0001$
No preference	2	3	4	2	
Prefer child to be gay or lesbian	1	9	0	0	

[a]Fisher's exact test p calculated for young adults from lesbian versus heterosexual mother families for "prefer child to be gay or lesbian" versus "no preference" or "prefer child to be heterosexual".
[b]Fisher's exact test p calculated for females from lesbian mother families versus females from heterosexual mother families for "prefer child to be gay or lesbian" versus "no preference," or "prefer child to be heterosexual" (Fisher's exact test $p = .006$). No significant difference for males of lesbian versus heterosexual mother families.

of contention (among other ongoing conflicts). The others felt that their mother's preference regarding their own sexual orientation neither influenced the development of their sexual identity nor adversely affected their relationship with her. Both Sara and her sister Tessa, daughters of a lesbian mother had only heterosexual relationships. Both have a close relationship with their mother and often talked to her about their boyfriends. Sara reported that her mother would tell her if she did not like her boyfriends. "But I would still have them round. She didn't mind. She was all right about them. . . . She just didn't allow them to stay overnight." Later in the same interview, Sara was asked whether she thought her mother prefered her to have lesbian relationships.

F. T.: Do you think she would prefer you to be a lesbian?

SARA: Well, I'm sure she would. I think she'd like it if me and Tessa were with women rather than men. In fact, I know Tessa's said she's talked about it with her. When Tessa's said she's had problems with her boyfriends, she said, "Why don't you try and see if you get on better with women?"

Heterosexual mothers were much less likely to discuss gay and lesbian relationships with their children. Of the 16 young people brought up by heterosexual mothers for whom data were available, six thought that their mother was tolerant of gay men and lesbian women, four had no idea what their mother's attitude was, and six reported that their mother's attitude was negative. It is interesting to note that Allen (1987) in her British survey of 14- to 16-year-olds found that only 7% of boys and 12% of girls remembered having discussed gay and lesbian relationships with their mother. For Anita, one of the interviewees brought up by a heterosexual mother in our study, her mother's reaction to her crush on a female teacher seemed to be influential in her dismissal of her attraction as being "nothing sexual."

F. T.: Can you remember your first crush?

ANITA: God, yes! My first crush was my teacher. I used to get teased mercilessly by my mum about it, and my mum's friend that lived across the road. Oh God, I was totally enthralled that someone could be so—not marvelous, but she knew so much, you see. She had so much information that I wanted to know, and I desperately wanted to know it all. I used to sit there and think, "Oh God, she's marvelous. She knows all this stuff." And I was besotted in an unhealthy sort of way. Nothing sexual in it.

F. T.: Did you feel she was attractive?

ANITA: Yeah, she was pretty, and I think that may have played a part in it. I just worshiped the ground that she walked on. The penny dropped one day, and I thought, "This is really unhealthy. She is just a teacher."

F. T.: Anything that made the penny drop?

ANITA: Yeah, my mum teasing me, saying, "How's your teacher again today?" I suddenly became aware that other people were noticing that I was walking round with my head in the clouds, and I thought, "Perhaps I can get a grip on myself."

Of the 25 interviewees from lesbian backgrounds, 11 felt that their mother had always been positive about their choice of partner, as did 12 of the 19 young people from heterosexual homes. For both groups of young people, their mother's acceptance of their partners appeared to be associated with the closeness of their relationship with her ($r = .530$, $p < .001$), and with her main partner ($r = .410$, $p = .007$). For young people from lesbian mother families, the mother's response to their partners was not associated with whether the young person had heterosexual or homosexual relationships.

PATTERNS OF RELATIONSHIP FORMATION

Data on the participants' relationship patterns were obtained to explore whether growing up in a lesbian mother family had an effect on the rate of adolescent sexual activity or on the type or quality of the relationships entered into. The first issue examined was whether young people from lesbian backgrounds have more or fewer sexual relationships than their peers from heterosexual homes. Previous studies and clinical case histories suggested that children with a lesbian or gay parent respond to their parent's sexual identity by increasing their involvement in heterosexual activity (B. Miller, 1979; K. G. Lewis, 1980; Javaid, 1983). However, as discussed in Chapter 2, increased relationship involvement may be attributable to the experience of parental separation and/or growing up in a father-absent household. It has been suggested that daughters of divorce, in particular, may be propelled into sexual relationships in an attempt to separate from the close preadolescent mother–daughter relationship that is often formed in father-absent households (Kalter, 1977; Kalter, Riemer, Brickman, & Chen, 1985; Wallerstein & Corbin, 1989).

Number and Timing of Sexual Relationships

For each interviewee, the total number of sexual partners from puberty to the time of follow-up was calculated and categorized according to the scale shown in Table 6.6. Although surveys of sexual behavior have simply counted the number of partners with whom the person has had vaginal intercourse (e.g., Knox, MacArthur, & Simons, 1993), we wished to include lesbian and gay relationships in our tally, and thus a less stringent criterion (genital touching) for both same-gender and opposite-gender relationships was used. As no one in the sample had experienced a same-gender sexual relationship prior to their first experience of vaginal in-

TABLE 6.6. Number of Sexual Relationships with Same-Gender and Opposite-Gender Partners Reported by Young Men and Women from Lesbian and Heterosexual Backgrounds

	Lesbian mother		Heterosexual mother[a]	
	Male	Female	Male	Female[b]
None	2	0	0	0
1	0	2	1	4
2–4	4	4	3	3
5–9	1	4	3	1
10–14	1	4	3	1
15–19	0	2	0	0

[a]Young adults from lesbian mother families versus young adults from heterosexual mother families ($t = .66$, $df = 41$, $p = $ NS).
[b]Females from lesbian mother families versus females from heterosexual mother families ($t = 2.23$, $df = 23$, $p < .05$).

tercourse, this point was considered to be the start of the young person's sexual career.

Young people from lesbian mother families and their counterparts from heterosexual homes reported similar numbers of sexual relationships, even when the two young men from lesbian mother families who reported no previous sexual relationships were excluded. The two groups of young people did not differ in age. However, when men and women were analyzed separately, young women from lesbian households reported a greater number of sexual relationships than did young women from heterosexual households ($t = 2.23$, $df = 23$, $p < .05$), indicating that gender and family background may interact. There was no significant difference between the number of sexual relationships reported by young men from the two types of family.

These findings are reasonably comparable to those reported in other British surveys of sexual behavior. Knox et al (1993) found the average number of sexual partners for participants aged 16 to 30 in their national questionnaire survey to be 6.5 for men and 3.5 for women. Taking the midpoint in each of our categories, the young men in our sample averaged slightly fewer relationships (5.5) and the young women more relationships (6.2) than did respondents in the survey by Knox et al. The percentage of young men in our follow-up study who reported five or more relationships (54%) is identical to Johnson and Wadsworth's

(1994) finding that 54% of men in the 16-to-34 age group reported five or more sexual partners in the British National Survey
of Sexual Attitudes and Lifestyles. However, 48% of the young
women in our study reported five or more sexual partners compared with only 33% of the young women aged 16 to 34 who
participated in the sexual attitudes and lifestyle survey. The greater
number of sexual relationships reported by young women in the
present study may reflect the adoption of a wider definition of
sexual relationships. In addition, the gender difference may have
arisen in response to being interviewed by a female interviewer.

To provide a more standard comparison with the majority
of surveys conducted on adolescents' sexual behavior, the respondents' age at first vaginal intercourse was also considered. Again,
there was no difference between young adults brought up by lesbian and heterosexual mothers ($t = .05$, $df = 40$, NS). The mean
age at which sexual intercourse first took place was 16.5 years.
Nor were there group differences when men and women were
analyzed separately. Wellings and Bradshaw (1994) reported that
for young people aged 16 to 24 in the British National Survey
of Sexual Attitudes and Lifestyles the median age at first intercourse was 17 years (excluding the 20% of 16- to 24-year-olds
who had not experienced heterosexual intercourse). Our findings also seem comparable with those quoted by Breakwell and
Fife-Schaw (1992) in their survey of over 2,000 16- to 20-year-
olds in southern England. They reported that about 55% of the
adolescent boys and girls surveyed had experienced vaginal intercourse by their 17th birthday. British adolescents tend to be
older than American adolescents when they begin their sexual
careers. For example, Moore and Erickson (1985) found that
the average age at first sexual intercourse among a sample of 16-
to 25-year-olds in Los Angeles, California, was 14.9 years for
boys and 15.9 years for girls.

Relationship Quality

Various indicators of the type and quality of relationships formed
by young people from lesbian and heterosexual mother families
were examined. Although the wide age range of interviewees
(from late teens to early 30s) presented difficulties for analyzing

data on relationship type for a small sample, the age range of the two groups was similar; thus, the groups were compared directly in terms of their current relationship status. Respondents were categorized according to three groups: those who were currently cohabiting (six people were married, and eight were living with their partner), those who were in a steady or committed relationship but were not living with the partner, and those who were currently single or who had occasional short-term relationships. Table 6.7 shows the current relationship status of interviewees from lesbian and heterosexual backgrounds. There was no significant difference in the proportions cohabiting or involved in a steady relationship between the lesbian and heterosexual mother family groups.

For interviewees who were currently involved in cohabiting and committed noncohabiting relationships, it was possible to examine their current satisfaction with and the extent of conflict within that relationship. No group difference was identified between interviewees from lesbian and heterosexual mother family backgrounds for either variable. In addition to the interview data, questionnaire data were gathered to obtain a measure of satisfaction with the current relationship that was independent of the interviewer's assessment. Young people who were currently married or cohabiting were asked to complete the Golombok–Rust Inventory of Marital Satisfaction (GRIMS), which discriminates between couples experiencing marital problems and a nonclinical population (Rust, Bennun, Crowe, & Golombok, 1988). With

TABLE 6.7. Young Adults' Current Relationship Status by Family Type

	Lesbian mother	Heterosexual mother	Fisher's exact p
No relationship	10	11	
			NS[a]
Noncohabiting steady relationship	8	2	
			NS[b]
Cohabiting (married or living with partner)	7	7	

[a]Fisher's exact test p calculated for "no relationship" versus "noncohabiting steady relationship" or "cohabiting relationship."
[b]Fisher's exact test p calculated for "no relationship" or "noncohabiting relationship" versus "cohabiting relationship."

respect to GRIMS norms for marital satisfaction, six of the seven young adults from lesbian mother families and five of the seven young adults from heterosexual family backgrounds obtained a score that indicated that their cohabiting relationship was above average or better. For example, Joshua (age 31 at the time of the follow-up study) had lived with his lesbian mother and her girlfriend until he was in his early twenties. He moved in with his girlfriend after they had been together for 6 months, and they had been living together for 4 years when he was interviewed.

JOSHUA: We met at this party, and it really was, I suppose, love at first sight. I remember saying, "She'll do for me." . . . We just hit it off rather quickly, and within a month we knew that we were right for each other. It went very quickly, and I was happy with her. There's been only once or twice when I thought, you know, "You've rushed into this," but carried on, you know. And it worked out well.

The numbers of interviewees from each type of family who had never cohabited, who were currently first-time cohabitees, who had previously cohabited once, and who had cohabited more than once in either a same-gender or opposite-gender relationship were examined. These data are shown separately for men and women in each group in Table 6.8. Over 60% of interviewees as a whole had cohabited at least once by the time of follow-up. Whether or not a young person had ever cohabited was not dependent upon his or her age at interview. However, the contrast between those who had never cohabited and those who had previously cohabited or were cohabiting at the time of the interview revealed that daughters were more likely to have cohabited than sons (Fisher's exact $p = .019$). There was no overall difference between young people from lesbian and heterosexual backgrounds in terms of their pattern of cohabitation. However, when men and women were analyzed separately, it was found that young women from lesbian mother families were more likely than the daughters of heterosexaul mothers to have finished their first cohabitation or to be involved in a subsequent cohabitation (Fisher's exact $p = .025$). Although young women from lesbian mother families may have had greater difficulty in maintaining a cohabit-

TABLE 6.8. Young Adults' Previous and Current Cohabitations
by Family Types

	Lesbian mother		Heterosexual mother		Fisher's
	Male	Female	Male	Female	exact *p*
Never cohabited	6	3	5	3	NS[a]
One current cohabitation	1	2	2	4	
One previous cohabitation	0	8	4	2	NS[b]
More than one cohabitation	1	4	0	0	

[a]Fisher's exact test *p* calculated for young adults from lesbian versus heterosexual mother families for never cohabited versus previously or currently cohabited.
[b]Fisher's exact test *p* calculated for young adults from lesbian versus heterosexual mother families for never or one current cohabitation versus one or more previous cohabitations.

ing relationship, an alternative explanation for this finding is that young women from lesbian backgrounds may be less likely to hold traditional ideas associating marriage or cohabitation with lifelong commitment.

Early partnerships in which young people move in together while still in their teens or marry or cohabit after only a brief relationship have been highlighted as particularly vulnerable to later strife and separation (Quinton & Rutter, 1988; Rutter, Quinton, & Hill, 1990; Kiernan, 1992). According to Rutter et al. (1990), partnerships are particularly vulnerable to difficulties if the young person is 18 or younger and if the couple have known each other for less than 6 months prior to living together. In examining our respondents according to these criteria, young people from lesbian backgrounds did not differ from their counterparts from heterosexual homes on age at first cohabitation or marriage. Furthermore, there was no significant difference between those from lesbian and heterosexual mother families in the length of time prior to cohabitation. However, compared with young women from heterosexual homes, young women from lesbian mother families decided to cohabit sooner: Compared to 1 out of 6 women from heterosexual backgrounds 10 out of 14 women from lesbian backgrounds cohabited after an initial relationship of less than 6 months (Fisher's exact $p = .021$). It is possible that daughters from lesbian mother families are more ready to experiment with relationships and hold less traditional ideas about cohabitation prior to marriage. For example, Sally left her mother and her mother's girlfriend's home when she was 18 years old because she wanted to pursue her relationship with her boyfriend.

SALLY: One night I met Steve, and I thought he was gorgeous! And then I wanted to go to bed with him, and his mum caught us on the way up to his bedroom. So he dropped me off at home, like, and that's when I wanted to move out so that I'd have more sexual freedom. And that's when I actually moved out of home.

Sally moved in with Steve, but their relationship ended after 2 years, partly because Sally had an affair with another man. When her relationship with Steve ended, Sally moved back home to her mother and her mother's girlfriend "just to get [herself] sorted out."

SUMMARY

Findings relating to the sexual orientation of children from lesbian mother families show that these young people are generally no more likely than their peers from heterosexual mother families to identify themselves as gay or lesbian or to be attracted to someone of the same gender. However, if they do experience same-gender attraction, they are more likely to pursue a sexual relationship. Young people from lesbian backgrounds are also more aware of the possibility of gay and lesbian relationships and perceive greater choice for themselves. In our study, the young adults from lesbian households in which there was greater openness about intimacy were the ones most likely to report same-gender sexual interest, although this may simply reflect their greater willingness to acknowledge gay and lesbian relationships.

Compared with heterosexual mothers, the lesbian mothers in our study generally were more able to communicate with their sons and daughters about adolescent sexual development and relationships. Young adults from lesbian backgrounds rarely felt that their mother had restricted the development of their sexual identity. In contrast, heterosexual mothers were unlikely to have considered that their children might have homosexual attractions and relationships. The intimate relationship patterns of our interviewees from lesbian mother families were generally similar to those exhibited by the comparison group of young men and women brought up by heterosexual mothers after their mother and father had separated. However, the young women from lesbian backgrounds seemed to be less bound by conservative norms restricting women's premarital sexual activity.

CHAPTER SEVEN

Psychological Adjustment

PERHAPS THE most common argument put forward by opponents of lesbian mother families is that children from these households will show poor psychological adjustment as a result of their upbringing and will continue to be troubled by mental health problems in adult life. The contention that these children will show poor psychological adjustment in childhood has not been supported by any of the investigations conducted so far (Patterson, 1992). Moreover, if the children of lesbian mothers do experience any emotional difficulties, these tend to resemble those of other children whose parents have divorced (K. G. Lewis, 1980; Kirkpatrick et al., 1981; Green et al., 1986). In the more general literature on the consequences of parental divorce, a small but significant difference is consistently observed between children from non-divorced families and children who have experienced parental separation, who show poorer psychological adjustment both in the short term (Amato & Keith, 1991a) and in the long term (Amato & Keith, 1991b). However, as discussed in Chapter 2, detrimental effects of parental separation on children's well-being appear to be largely mediated by continued family conflict, deteriorating parent–child relationships, and reduced socioeconomic status rather than by parental separation per se (Emery, 1988; Hetherington & Camara, 1988).

Although there is no evidence to suggest that upbringing in a lesbian household itself is associated with an increased risk of psychological problems in childhood, little is known about possible outcomes in adolescence or adulthood. It has been suggested that psychological difficulties may only emerge during

adolescence, when the young person begins to form intimate relationships and becomes more aware of prejudice against lesbian
women and gay men. Similar "sleeper effects" have been suggested
in the divorce literature (Wallerstein & Corbin, 1989). However,
the only existing study of lesbian mother families examined the
self-esteem of adolescents and did not find detrimental effects
(Huggins, 1989).

ANXIETY, DEPRESSION,
AND PSYCHIATRIC CONTACT

The long-term psychological effects of upbringing in a lesbian
mother family were assessed in the present study both by questionnaire and by interview. During the interview, the young people were asked to complete two questionnaire measures of
emotional well-being, the Trait Anxiety Inventory (Spielberger,
1983) and the Beck Depression Inventory (Beck & Steer, 1987),
to assess current levels of anxiety and depression, respectively.
For both inventories, the higher the score the more severe the
symptoms. Both of these measures have been shown to have good
reliability and to discriminate well between clinical and nonclinical groups.

Interview data were also obtained on whether the young person had ever experienced episodes of anxiety or depression for
which help had been sought from a health care professional (medical doctor, psychologist, counselor, or therapist) and on whether
he or she had ever consulted a medical doctor about various psychosomatic indicators of stress (e.g., sleep problems or alcohol,
cigarette, or drug consumption). This information formed the
basis for rating the dichotomous variable "professional consultation for mental health problem."

Results shown in Table 7.1 indicate no significant difference between participants from lesbian and heterosexual homes
for the Trait Anxiety Inventory. The scores of young adults from
both types of family background were closely comparable to the
norms for working males and females aged 19 to 39 in the United States (Spielberger, 1983). Similarly, the groups did not differ
on level of depression as assessed by the Beck Depression Inven-

TABLE 7.1. Young Adults' Depression and Anxiety Scores by Family Type

	Group	Mean	SD	t	df	p
Trait Anxiety Inventory	Lesbian mother	41.36	10.84	.95	41	NS
	Heterosexual mother	38.38	9.58			
Beck Depression Inventory	Lesbian mother	8.21	6.11	.60	43	NS
	Heterosexual mother	7.24	4.56			

tory. When the cutoff point of 15, recommended by Frank et al. (1991) to indicate the presence of depressive symptomatology, was used, no group difference emerged between the proportions of young adults categorized as depressed (see Table 7.2). In addition, a similar proportion of interviewees from each type of family reported contact with health care professionals in connection with problems arising from anxiety, depression, or stress.

Of the nine young adults from lesbian mother families who reported mental health problems, seven reported that they had consulted a mental health professional for anxiety or depression and two had attempted suicide. Similarly, of the seven young adults from heterosexual mother families who had consulted a health professional for mental health problems, four had experienced feelings of anxiety or depression, one had previously attempted suicide, and two had a history of substance abuse. There was no statistically significant difference between the groups with respect to type of mental health problem reported. One of the young men from a heterosexual family background who declined to participate in the study was at that time receiving psychiatric care for schizophrenia.

Interviewees were asked what events or reasons they connected with the onset of their mental health problem. None of the interviewees from lesbian or heterosexual mother families recalled difficulties in family relationships precipitating a consultation for a mental health problem, except for one daughter of a heterosexual mother who mentioned problems in her relationship with her mother and stepfather as a possible cause of her distress. For young adults from both lesbian and heterosexual mother families, difficulties in intimate relationships were the

TABLE 7.2. Number of Young Adults Seeking Professional Consultations for Psychological Problems and Scoring above Cutoff on the Beck Depression Inventory by Family Type

		Lesbian mother	Heterosexual mother	Fisher's exact *p*
Psychological problems	Professional consultation	9	7	NS
	No problems	16	14	
Beck Depression Inventory	Score greater than or equal to 15	4	2	NS
	Score less than or equal to 14	21	19	

Note. From Tasker and Golombok (1995). Copyright 1995 by the American Orthopsychiatric Association, Inc. Reprinted by permission.

common problems reported for the period prior to seeking professional help. Patti attributed her need for antidepressants to the negative impact of life events since her divorce a year earlier, and to the stress of a new relationship. Like others in the study, Patti thought that her mother had been supportive through her difficulties.

F. T.: I'm asking everybody who is involved in the project if they've ever felt anxious or depressed.

PATTI: Yeah, this year, about a month ago. Well, maybe a bit longer than that. I was really depressed. . . . I went to the doctors when I realized eventually, when I realized that if I didn't do something about it that I was going to destroy everything else in my life. 'Cause I was ruining things with me and [new boyfriend] because I was so terrible to live with. But, um, all he did was prescribe me with antidepressants.

F. T.: Have you had any other spells of anxiety or depression?

PATTI: Only with my marriage, really. . . . I got quite ill during the marriage because it was just so much strain on me. . . . I think that the reason for the depression this time has been the last years . . . just sort of building up and up and up and always coping, coping. . . . I think it all just— and with the divorce and changing jobs and, you know, there's a lot of stressful things happening all at one go and a new relationship. . . . So I think it was just a combination of everything.

EMPLOYMENT HISTORY

Data on career history provide another indicator of well-being in adulthood, since employment difficulties are often associated with poor psychological adjustment. Conversely, periods of unemployment may contribute to poor mental health (Goldberg & Huxley, 1992). All interviewees were asked for their age at the time they left the education system and for the highest qualification they had obtained so far. They were then asked to give a chronological history of their employment (and periods of unemployment) since leaving school and their reasons for leaving previous jobs. Those who were rated as currently experiencing employment difficulties had all been unemployed for at least a year and none was actively seeking employment at the time of follow-up. The economic recession in Britain in the early 1990s meant that many of the young people who took part in the study had experienced periods of unemployment.

No significant difference was found between young adults from lesbian versus heterosexual mother families in terms of their employment history (see Table 7.3). There was no difference between women from the two family types with respect to employment history. However, a nonsignificant trend (Fisher's exact $p = .051$) in the data suggested that more men from heterosexual backgrounds were currently unemployed (5/12) than men from lesbian mother families (0/8). This finding may be attributable to the larger proportion of interviewees of working-class origin in the heterosexual family group.

CHILDHOOD CHARACTERISTICS OF ADULTS REPORTING MENTAL HEALTH PROBLEMS

Whereas young adults brought up by lesbian mothers appeared to generally continue to have good psychological adjustment and were no more likely to experience mental health problems than

TABLE 7.3. Employment Histories of Young Adults Raised in Lesbian and Heterosexual Mother Families

	Lesbian mother		Heterosexual mother		Fisher's exact p^a
	Male	Female	Male	Female	
Consistent career success	2	4	3	5	
Currently in college	3	2	2	0	NS
Previous employment problems	3	5	2	2	
Current employment problems	0	5	5	1	

Note. Two young women (one from a lesbian mother family and one from a heterosexual mother family) were excluded from this table because their employment history had been affected by bringing up their own children.
^{a}Fisher's exact test p calculated for data on men and women combined for previous or current experience of employment problems versus consistent career success or currently in college.

their peers from families headed by heterosexual mothers, in both groups of families a few individuals reported psychological problems at some time during adolescence or early adulthood. We now examine which childhood experiences were associated with mental health difficulties among young adults from lesbian and heterosexual mother families.

Previous research indicates that various childhood experiences may have an adverse impact on long-term emotional well-being. Huggins (1989) reported that daughters of lesbian mothers tend to have poorer self-esteem if they hold a negative attitude toward their mother's lesbian identity, if their father does not accept their mother's lesbian identity, and if they learn about their mother's lesbian relationships during their adolescent years. Huggins (1989) also found that adolescents from both lesbian and heterosexual mother families who live with a mother who is on her own tend to have lower self-esteem than those living with a mother and her partner.

Research on the quality of heterosexual stepfamily relationships for both stepmother and stepfather families has found that residential parent–stepparent relationship satisfaction is associated with more positive stepparent–stepchild relationships and better psychological adjustment among stepsons but not stepdaughters (Brand, Clingempeel, & Bowen-Woodward, 1988). It has also been found that after parental divorce children show optimal psychological adjustment when socioeconomic resources do not diminish, when the child's relationships with both residential and nonresidential parents remain good, and when mothers and fathers achieve amicable postdivorce parenting arrangements (Hetherington & Camara, 1988).

Other childhood circumstances have also been related to mental health problems in adult life. Parental mental illness is associated with an increased likelihood of mental health problems among children, and children with emotional and behavioral problems are more likely to experience mental health difficulties in adulthood (Rutter & Madge, 1976). An association between poor peer relationships in childhood and later adult psychopathology has also been described (Parker & Asher, 1987).

Table 7.4 displays point biserial correlations between variables from the original study and whether or not the interviewee reported consulting a health professional for mental health difficulties; these analyses are presented separately for young adults from lesbian and heterosexual mother families. Similarly, Table 7.5 shows point biserial correlations between followup study variables and professional consultation for mental health problems; again, these analyses are presented separately for the two groups of young adults.

For young adults from a lesbian mother family background, a significant association was found between the mother's experience of psychiatric care in the year prior to the original study and the interviewee's report of mental health problems ($r = .577$, $p < .01$; see Table 7.4). In addition, the children of lesbian mothers whose mothers had higher scores on the Malaise Inventory of psychosomatic symptoms (Rutter et al., 1970) at the time of the original study were more likely to have consulted a professional for psychological problems in adulthood ($r = .492$, $p < .05$). Whether they had been separated from their lesbian mother for at least a month during their childhood also showed a nonsignificant trend toward an association with later mental health problems ($r = .393$, $p < .10$). However, if their mother had

TABLE 7.4. Correlations between Childhood Family Characteristics and Young Adults' Reports of Consultation with a Mental Health Professional

	Lesbian mother	Heterosexual mother
Mother's and child's psychological adjustment at the time of the initial study		
Mother's contact with psychiatric services ever (0, "never"–1, "contact with psychiatric services")	–.067 (24)	.676*** (19)
Mother's contact with psychiatric services in *the year prior to study* (0, "none"–1, "contact with psychiatric services")	.577** (24)	.409† (19)
Mother's Malaise Inventory Score (0, "score below 7"–1, "score 7 and above")	.492* (25)	–.224 (21)
Child's Rutter A Scale Score (mother's report) (0, "score below 13"–1, "score 13 and above")	.086 (25)	–.086 (21)
Child's Rutter B Scale Score (teacher's report) (0, "score below 9"–1, "score 9 and above")	–.019 (17)	.150 (17)
Family relationships at time of initial study		
Mother's expressed warmth to child (0, "none"–5, "very warm")	.091 (24)	–.071 (20)
Child separated from mother prior to initial study (0, "no separations"–1, "separated")	.393† (25)	.172 (21)
Mother's relationship history (0, "4 partners or fewer"–1, "more than four partners or concurrent relationships")	–.164 (25)	—
Quality of mother's relationship with her female partner (1, "fully harmonious"–5, "serious conflict")	–.425 (13)	—
Mother and partner share child care (0, "mother and partner share"–1, "mother main caregiver")	–.365 (13)	—
Child's contact with father (0, "none"–2, "at least weekly")	–.177 (25)	–.139 (21)
Number of years child raised in heterosexual home	.085 (25)	—
Peers' response at time of initial study		
Quality of child's peer relationships (0, "good"–2, "definite difficulties")	.083 (19)	–.234 (20)

† $p < .10$; * $p < .05$; ** $p < .01$; *** $p < .001$.

TABLE 7.5. Correlations between Family Characteristics Assessed at Follow-Up and Young Adults' Reports of Consultation with a Mental Health Professional

	Lesbian mother	Heterosexual mother
Family relationships at follow-up		
Current relationship with mother	.184	−.412†
(1, "very negative"–4, "very positive")	(25)	(21)
Adolescent relationship with mother's partner	−.149	−.744***
(1, "very negative"–4, "very positive")	(24)	(20)
Current relationship with mother's partner	.141	−.361
(1, "very negative"–4, "very positive")	(24)	(17)
Mother's relationship style	.010	−.074
(1, "exclusive"–4, "nonexclusive")	(24)	(20)
Conflict in mother's primary relationship	.118	−.083
(1, "regular episodes of conflict"–	(22)	(20)
4, "no serious conflict")		
Feelings about family identity during adolescence	.133	−.018
(1, "very negative"–4, "very positive")	(24)	(20)
Feelings about family identity as a young adult	.127	−.075
(1, "very negative"–4, "very positive")	(24)	(19)
Closeness of current relationship with father	.019	.057
(1, "very negative"–4, "very positive")	(19)	(13)
Father's attitude toward mother's relationships	.408	.108
(1, "opposed/upset"–3, "expressed support")	(17)	(11)
Peers' response at follow-up		
Teased about mother's lifestyle	−.042	.289
(0, "not teased"–1, "teased about mother")	(25)	(21)
Teased about own sexuality	−.161	.172
(0, "not teased"–1, "teased about sexuality")	(25)	(21)

† $p < .10$; *** $p < .001$.

experienced psychiatric care, they were more likely to have been separated from her, suggesting that separation from mother is not an independent effect.

For young adults from heterosexual mother families, mothers' histories of psychiatric problems also appeared to be related to those of their adult children. Table 7.4 shows that heterosexual mothers' reports of psychiatric contact, either immediately prior to the initial study or earlier, were correlated with reports of adult mental health problems among their offspring ($r = .409, p < .10$, and $r = .676, p < .001$, respectively). The relationship between maternal psychiatric history and an interviewee's mental health problems in early adulthood thus appears to be a general effect operating independently of the mother's sexual orientation. This longitudinal association between psychological well-being and maternal mental health is congruent with more general research on the intergenerational transmission of psychological disorder.

Follow-up study variables measuring the quality of family relationships were correlated with the presence of mental health problems among young adults from heterosexual mother families (see Table 7.5). For these young men and women, the experience of mental health problems was associated with a poor relationship with their stepfather ($r = -.744, p < .001$) and also showed a nonsignificant trend toward an association with a poor relationship with their mother ($r = -.412, p < .10$). These correlations were not found to be statistically significant for lesbian mother families, perhaps because interviewees from lesbian backgrounds generally reported better relationships with their mother's female partner (see Chapter 4).

Unlike the study by Huggins (1989), the present study revealed no evidence in either group of participants for an association between interviewees' psychological well-being and either the quality of their relationship with their father or their father's response to their mother's new relationships. Furthermore, no relationship was found between young adults' attitude toward their mother's sexual identity and their general emotional well-being. Nor was there evidence for a link between poor peer relationships in childhood and later mental health problems for the young adults from either group.

SUMMARY

In our study, men and women raised by lesbian mothers were no more likely than their peers from heterosexual homes to experience anxiety or depression. The scores for both groups of young adults on the depression and anxiety inventories fell within the normal range. Furthermore, young adults from lesbian mother families were no more likely than those from heterosexual backgrounds to have sought professional help for mental health problems.

In concordance with previous research on the childhood correlates of adult mental health, we found maternal psychiatric history to be associated with mental health problems among the young adults who reported contact with mental health services. This was so irrespective of the mother's sexual orientation. Only for young adults from heterosexual mother families was there any evidence that those who reported mental health problems also remembered a more difficult relationship with their stepparent.

CHAPTER EIGHT

Conclusions

W HAT DO young people think about the experience of growing up in a lesbian mother family? Over one-third of the young adults who had been brought up by a lesbian mother were proud of her sexual identity. Reflecting on their earlier feelings as adolescents, 38% reported that they had accepted the fact that their mother was having a lesbian relationship and had not attempted to keep their family background secret from close friends. However, most remembered feeling some concern about peer prejudice, and many were cautious about telling others about their family. Children brought up by a lesbian mother not only showed good adjustment in personal and social development as young children but also continued to function well as adolescents and as young adults, experiencing no detrimental long-term effects in terms of their mental health, their family relationships, and relationships with peers and partners in comparison with those from heterosexual mother families.

Before proceeding to discuss the implications of our study, it is necessary to consider whether it is reasonable to generalize from the findings presented here to paint a broader picture of the well-being of young adults raised in lesbian mother families. It was obviously not feasible to recruit a general population sample of lesbian mothers, given that many do not publicly declare their sexual identity. In the original study, volunteers were contacted through various lesbian publications and groups; thus, the mothers who volunteered may have been different in some way from other lesbian mothers (although similar procedures were used to recruit the heterosexual single mothers to control for self-selection biases). Nevertheless, it remains unknown how representative the sample was for lesbian and single heterosexual mothers as a whole. Both the lesbian and the heterosexual mother groups reflected a fair diversity of families nationwide; subjects were from different socioeconomic backgrounds and held different political perspectives. It can be argued that the young adults from both types of family were atypical in comparison to their counterparts raised in heterosexual homes with both mother and father present. Although this possibility cannot be refuted, the results have been placed in the context of established population norms where these are available.

Interview data are always open to criticisms of bias owing to self-presentation effects. Indeed, it is reasonable to suspect that lesbian mothers may wish to portray an overly positive picture of family life in view of the discrimination they often face in a predominantly heterosexual society. However, this motivation may apply less to the children than to the mothers themselves. Nevertheless, steps were taken to minimize this potential source of bias. The flexible semistructured interview schedule enabled the interviewer to probe any apparently contradictory answers that arose in response to similar questions on the same issue, and the in-depth, open-ended approach allowed interviewees to register any dissatisfaction they might have had with their upbringing.

A major strength of this research is the use of prospective data gathered from interviews with the mothers *before* the long-term outcomes for the children were known. These data are therefore independent of the young person's retrospective interpretation of events. Furthermore, the young people contacted for follow-up were not invited to participate in the study on the basis of adult outcome. In the main, the young people who accepted our invitation to participate in the follow-up study were not notably different from those we were unable to interview for the longitudinal study. However, as we discussed in Chapter 3, there are a couple of indications that we may have lost from the follow-up study those young people from lesbian mother families who were less aware of their mother's having a lesbian relationship at the time of the original study and those whose mothers were less happy in their cohabiting relationship at that point. Thus, the positive long-term findings from the follow-up study may reflect the views of young people whose mothers were more open with them and who had grown up in a happy family environment. However, within the follow-up sample of young adults from lesbian mother families we were able to explore whether differences in the quality of early family environment did contribute to key long-term outcomes.

Although any major effects of upbringing in a lesbian household are likely to have been identified in the present study, subtle differences between the two types of family may not have been detected owing to the small sample size. This was particularly problematic when investigating possible sex and social class differences between young women and men brought up in lesbian and heterosexual homes. Because of the low statistical power, nonsignificant trends within the data were reported. Particular caution is obviously required in generalizing from these results.

THE MAIN FINDINGS

From a legal and public policy perspective, a key finding is that children from lesbian mother families continue to have good mental health in adulthood. Young people from lesbian mother families in our study were no more likely than those from heterosexual family backgrounds to have sought professional help for mental health problems. Likewise, they were no more likely to be anxious or depressed at follow-up. Congruent with the wider literature on developmental psychopathology, young adults who had experienced mental health problems from either type of family background were those whose mothers had reported poor mental health at the time of the original study. This was found to be the case, irrespective of the mother's sexual orientation.

When asked about their family relationships, young people from lesbian mother families reported more positive relationships with their mother's female partner, both as adults and during adolescence, than did the young adults from heterosexual mother families who reported on their relationship with their mother's new male partner. However, it is important to remember that the comparisons between follow-up participants and nonparticipants indicated that the sample may have lost children from lesbian mother families whose mothers reported less positive relationships with their female partner. Mothers' female partners could perhaps more easily be added to the family in the role of a "second mum." These findings suggest that greater public and legal recognition should be given to the importance of child's relationship with the mother's female partner. Furthermore, these findings relating to lesbian postdivorce families challenge the conclusions drawn from previous research on heterosexual stepfamilies concerning the difficulties of stepmother–stepchild relationships.

Young people from lesbian mother families generally enjoyed good relationships with their mother and their nonresident father. There were no significant differences between young adults from the two family types, for either daughters or sons, in their recollections of the quality of their mother's main relationship while they were living at home. The good family relationships reported by the young adults raised by lesbian mothers, together with the findings on their long-term well-being, indicate that these factors are unaffected by maternal sexual orientation.

The mother's reports of the quality of family relationships in the original study were generally not associated with how the young people felt about coming from a lesbian mother family. In some families much had happened in the intervening years. Therefore, in many ways it is not surprising that there are limited effects of early experience. Furthermore, it was mothers who reported on family life in the original study whereas children's impressions were the focus of the follow-up; the young people had obviously experienced family life somewhat differently from their mothers. However, if their mother had a stable, long-term lesbian relationship at the time of the original study, young people were more likely to be accepting of their family background during adolescence. It seems reasonable to suggest that the stability of their mother's main adult relationship matters to children, irrespective of the mother's sexual orientation. However, there is no equivalent prospective data on the relationship history of the heterosexual mothers to establish this point, since all were single at the time of the original study. Just as with heterosexual stepfamilies, a stable parental relationship may make it easier for young people to accept their family situation, perhaps because there is no need to reexamine changes in family composition.

Children are teased or bullied for all sorts of reasons, but the present findings indicate that young adults from lesbian mother families are no more likely than those from heterosexual backgrounds to report having been picked on by classmates. However, in our study there was a slight tendency for young people brought up by a lesbian mother to be more likely than those from heterosexual mother families to remember having been teased about their own sexuality. This appeared to be particularly true for boys. This may reflect the fact that children from lesbian mother families are indeed more likely to be teased about being lesbian or gay themselves, or it may mean that such children are more sensitive to name calling because it strikes a chord and that this sensitivity makes them more likely to remember such incidents.

In our study, over half of the young people from lesbian mother families were able to inform at least one close friend about their family who did not react negatively or tell others. Furthermore, young people from lesbian mother families were no more likely than those from heterosexual mother families to report difficulty in bringing friends home. However, about a third of the young people from lesbian mother families did think that their mother had been too open about her sexual identity in front of their school friends, an opinion that reflects their concern about peers unwittingly finding out about their family background. As a group, the children from lesbian mother families generally continued to experience good peer relationships, as recorded in the original study, and were able to integrate friends and family as they progressed through adolescence. Perhaps because they were generally alert to the possibility of homophobia, most mothers were able to assist their children in avoiding prejudice.

Those young adults who were negative or embarrassed about coming from a lesbian mother family during their adolescent years, and even into adulthood, were more likely to remember being teased at school, particularly about their own sexual identity. The experience of peer group stigmatization may therefore have had a negative effect on children's own attitudes toward the family, although it is also possible that children with a negative attitude toward their family may have suffered more from peer group discrimination. Young people from lesbian mother families who felt less accepting of their family during adolescence were also more likely to believe that their mother had been too open about her own sexual identity in front of their school friends and were more likely to have found it difficult to bring either school friends or partners home to meet their family. This suggests that fear of peer group stigmatization and the experience of being teased or bullied are central elements in how children feel about growing up in a lesbian mother family.

In disputed custody cases, concern is still expressed about the possibility that children will suffer the consequences of peer group stigmatization if they are brought up by lesbian parents who are "out" in the local community and active in lesbian politics. The present findings suggest no negative effects of the mother's involvement in lesbian or gay organizations. If anything, the data suggest that young people who became proud of their family tended to be those whose mothers were out at the time of the original study and involved in feminist issues or in lesbian or gay rights politics. Furthermore, the young person's experience of peer group stigmatization during adolescence did not appear to be influenced by the mother's involvement in lesbian or feminist politics but was instead influenced by whether or not the child's peers were welcomed at home.

The commonly held assumption that boys and girls brought up in a lesbian mother family will grow up to have a gay or lesbian sexual identity as adults is not supported by the findings of this study. There was no difference between the proportions of young adults from lesbian and heterosexual mother families who reported at least one instance of same-gender sexual attraction. However, compared with those from heterosexual mother families, young adults from lesbian mother families were more likely to have considered the possibility of having a lesbian or gay relationship and to have had a relationship with someone of the same gender if they felt attracted to them. Nevertheless, the finding that 23 out of 25 young adults from lesbian mother families identified as heterosexual in early adulthood indicates that consideration of or even involvement in a homosexual relationship does not necessarily lead to a homosexual or bisexual identity.

What do the findings reveal about the processes of sexual identity formation? Since the mothers and children who participated in the follow-up study were all genetically related to each other, it cannot be ruled out that the greater interest in same-gender sexual relationships shown by the children of lesbian mothers was due to biological influences rather than to upbringing or social factors or to an interaction between the two. It was beyond the scope of this study to evaluate any biological contribution. However, the variations among the young people from lesbian mother families in terms of their upbringing and their experience of same-gender attraction and relationships suggest that sexual orientation is influenced to some extent by the social environment in which children grow up. It seems that the experience of same-gender relationships may be more influenced by social factors than either the experience of same-gender attraction or the longer-term development of a bisexual or homosexual identity. The findings indicate that a family environment in which a mother is more open about her relationships with other women and does not express a preference for her child to necessarily have heterosexual relationships enables a young person to become involved in a homosexual relationship if the young person feels attracted to someone of the same sex. In our study, daughters of lesbian mothers were more likely than daughters of heterosexual mothers to have considered the possibility of a lesbian relationship or to have gone ahead and had a relationship with another woman. The fact that young women rather than young men from lesbian mother families were more willing to enter into same-gender relationships may be explained by the more obvious parallel with their mother's situation (and the small number of men from lesbian mother families in the sample may mean that the implications for sons in lesbian mother families went undetected).

The findings from our study are congruent with social cognitive theories of gender development, which suggest that children do not simply model parental behavior but first evaluate its suitability through their increasing awareness of the cultural appropriateness of the behavior. Where there has been an openness about and acceptance of lesbian relationships in the family environment, the young person growing up in a lesbian mother family is able to consider lesbian or gay relationships as a viable option whereas the dominant heterosexual culture ignores or denigrates homosexual relationships. Similarly, social constructionist theories emphasize that the sexual scripts that influence relationship formation are widened by a person's increasing knowledge of lesbian and gay subcultures. Furthermore, the association between young people's reports of their mother's involvement in feminist politics and their own experience of same-gender attraction and relationships suggests that when lesbian mothers endorse a political analysis of gender relationships within society, their children are more likely to develop a broader view of sexual relationships themselves.

The following case history illustrates the main findings from this study. At the time of the follow-up study Ben was 20, had experienced no mental health problems, and was currently studying for a degree in humanities. While this particular case history was selected because Ben articulated many of the issues expressed by young adults with lesbian mothers, Ben's family background was unusual in our sample in that he had never known his father.

Ben was brought up by his mother, and can not remember his mother having had a relationship with his father. His mother has had two consecutive cohabiting relationships with female partners (Irma and Joanne) through Ben's childhood and adolescence. Ben reported good relationships with both Irma and Joanne: "Joanne made me feel really welcome and integrated, so it was really good." Ben was more neutral in his feelings toward his mother's current noncohabiting partner, Georgina: "I think she's all right. It's just you don't mesh all the time, I suppose."

From age 12 through most of his high school years, Ben experienced intermittent teasing from his school peers, partly about matters unrelated to his family background but also about his mother's lesbian identity and briefly about his own sexuality. He recalled: "I wasn't, you know, accused of being gay or anything myself. I mean, I think there was a tiny time when I think I was. It was basically just trying to put up with jibes about my mum."

When asked for further details about these incidents, Ben replied: "They didn't even know what they were saying because it was just rumors that my mum was a lesbian and they were just saying it for a laugh. Like they'd say it to everyone—"Oh, your mum's a lesbian"—you know. But I didn't actually disagree. . . . I just sort of stayed silent." Irrespective of peer group stigma, Ben was able to make "quite a few good friends at school." By his last year of high school some students even thought his family was "really cool." "It's great! Hey, your mum's a lesbian! Wow!" . . . Because [by then] everyone was more aware or open."

Ben reported that all his sexual experiences have been with women, that he first experienced heterosexual intercourse at age 16, and that since then he has had two other full sexual relationships (one of which lasted a year). His mother welcomed all his girlfriends. Ben saw himself as heterosexual, although he reported having thought about relationships with men: " I mean, I think I still do, or I have had, fantasies with blokes. Not that I fancy a bloke, but sometimes you see a bloke in the street and you think he's attractive enough to go out with, he's the kind of bloke that you'd really like to go out with, even though you're not in the least gay. . . . But it's, you know, female-based fantasies mainly."

Ben's general attitude toward growing up in a lesbian mother family changed during adolescence: "Sometimes when I was growing up, it was, like, embarrassingly open, you know. It was, like, "Okay, Mum, you know why you're a lesbian, why you are what you are, but you don't need to blab about it so much, you know." I mean, this is only when I was young, you know." Ben reported that he is now much more upfront in telling others about his family background: "I make a point of telling everyone because it's not like you hide that you've got a dad. So why should I hide that my mum's got a girlfriend, you know. I don't, obviously, initially say, "Hello, my name's Ben, and my mother's a lesbian!" You know, I don't blurt it out in the first couple of sentences, but I'll make a point of telling people. Because there's no point in hiding it away; because it only makes it worse. You know, makes it seem more underground, [indiscreet], or terrible if you hide it away."

BEYOND THE LONGITUDINAL STUDY

Any longitudinal study is positioned within its historical context, and the social milieu in which lesbian mothers are bringing up their children has altered considerably over recent decades. Prior to the women's movement and the lesbian and gay liberation campaigns of the late 1960s, mothers who had relationships with other women would rarely have identified themselves as lesbian to the outside world. The majority would have accommodated (with more or less dissatisfaction) to bringing up children within marriage. The growing number of openly gay and lesbian men and women, the general increase in the acceptability of divorce, and the economic feasibility for women of living independently of men has enabled increasing numbers of lesbian mothers to make the decision to bring up their children outside of marriage and with their female partner.

The present study, begun in the mid-1970s, reflects this process. In the lesbian mother family group, all but one of the young adults who were followed up had lived with their mother and father for at least a year after their birth. Therefore, the group is essentially one of children of divorce growing up in a lesbian mother family. The study raises particular issues concerning the role of the nonresidential father and relationships within stepfamilies. Compared with children born into a lesbian mother family from the outset, or adopted by a single lesbian woman or a lesbian couple, the children in our study experienced the transition from a heterosexual family to a lesbian mother family, a transition that may well be a difficult one to adjust to. Not only did these children see their father leave and their mother explore relationships with women, but they also needed to build a relationship with their mother's new partner. The visibility of the family, and the potential for attracting prejudice, may also be influenced by the mother's late entry into lesbian relationships.

Finally, the implications for sexual orientation for children from postdivorce lesbian mother families may be different from those for children born into lesbian mother families. Since every lesbian mother of a young person in our follow-up study had had an earlier relationship with a man, it could be argued that these women all had a bisexual rather than a homosexual orientation (although the majority would not necessarily describe themselves in this way). Furthermore, if psychoanalytic theories are correct in arguing that early family environment is crucial for later sexual orientation, then the early years in a heterosexual family may have influenced the sexual identity of the young people we studied from postdivorce lesbian mother families in a heterosexual direction. However, the association found in our study of lesbian mother families between the degree of openness and acceptance of lesbian and gay relationships and the young people's experience of same-gender relationships indicates that it is family attitudes, either as accepting or rejecting of gay and lesbian relationships, that influence the young person's same-gender sexual interest. This process may operate independently of whether the child is raised in a lesbian mother family from birth or is born to a woman who is in a heterosexual relationship and subsequently identifies herself as lesbian. It is also important to remember that the young adults in the follow-up study were born at a time when there was less social acceptance of lesbian women and gay men than is true today. As Gagnon (1990) has pointed out, young people are now better informed about lesbian and gay cultures and know about lesbian and gay possibilities at an earlier age. It is conceivable that children born at the present time to heterosexual parents who are accepting of lesbian and gay relationships will be just as open to same-sex exploration in adulthood as the young adults from lesbian mother families are today. How the changing social climate will influence not only young people's exploration of same-gender relationships but also the general acceptance of lesbian mother families remains open to speculation.

What is clear from the present study is that it is not necessarily the case that children who are raised in a lesbian mother family will experience difficulties in adulthood. Indeed, the findings from the present study show that young people brought up by a lesbian mother do well in adulthood and have good relationships with their family, friends, and partners. In policy decisions about who should and should not be allowed to raise children, negative outcomes for children should not be assumed on the basis of a mother's sexual orientation.

1976–1977 Study Interviews with Mothers and Children: Variables Used in the Statistical Analyses

Child's gender

Child's age

Child's age when mother and father separated

Number of years child spent in a heterosexual family before mother identified herself as lesbian

Mother's educational qualifications
  0 = No college education
  1 = College education

Mother's occupational status (Registrar General's assignment of social class)
  0 = Not working
  1 = Middle class (I, II, and III nonmanual occupation)
  2 = Working class (III manual occupation, IV, and V)

Mother's previous use of psychiatric services
  0 = None
  1 = Mother previously under psychiatric care with her family doctor or a psychiatric hospital

Mother's use of psychiatric services in the year prior to original study
  0 = None
  1 = Mother under psychiatric care with her family doctor or a psychiatric hospital

Mother's Malaise Inventory score
  0 = Score below cutoff point of 7, indicating no psychiatric difficulties
  1 = Score of 7 or above, indicating possible psychiatric problems

Mother's rating of child's emotional and behavioral problems on Rutter A2 scale
  0 = Score below cutoff point of 13 indicating no psychiatric difficulties
  1 = Score of 13 or above indicating possible psychiatric problems

Child's schoolteacher's rating of child's emotional and behavioral problems on Rutter B2 scale
  0 = Score below cutoff point of 9, indicating no psychiatric difficulties
  1 = Score of 9 or above, indicating possible psychiatric problems

Mother's report of child's contact with father prior to original study
  0 = None
  1 = Less than weekly
  2 = At least once a week

Mother's expressed warmth to child (interviewer's rating over entire interview of mother's positive feelings toward child, based on spontaneity, tone of voice, expression, and gesture when talking about child; sympathy and concern for and empathy with child; and interest in the child as a person)
  0 = No demonstration of warmth to child (distant)
  1 = Little warmth
  2 = Some warmth
  3 = Moderate warmth
  4 = Moderately high warmth
  5 = High warmth

Child's separation from mother for a period of over a month prior to original study
  0 = No
  1 = Yes

Quality of child's peer relationships as reported by mother
  0 = Good
  1 = Slight difficulties only
  2 = Definite difficulties

Mother and child's report of child's gender role (combined scale); from low score indicating gender-typed behavior to extremely cross-gendered behavior

VARIABLES MEASURED ONLY
FOR LESBIAN MOTHER FAMILIES

Quality of lesbian mother's cohabiting relationship
1 = Fully harmonious
2 = Generally harmonious
3 = No serious conflict
4 = Substantial conflict
5 = Serious conflict

Extent to which lesbian mother and her partner share child care
0 = Partner is main caregiver, or child care is shared equally
1 = Mother is main caregiver

Mother's relationship style prior to original study
0 = Four or fewer monogamous relationships over the previous 5 years
1 = Five or more relationships in the previous 5 years or concurrent affairs

Mother's openness in expressing physical affection to her partner in front of child
0 = None
1 = Greeting kiss or hug
2 = Kiss or caress

Mother's contentment with her sexual identity
1 = Prefers to be heterosexual
2 = Probably would have preferred to be heterosexual
3 = Neutral
4 = Positive about lesbian identity but some difficulties experienced with it
5 = Positive about lesbian identity

Mother "out" about her lesbian identity in her local community (colleagues at work, neighbors and acquaintances)
0 = No
1 = Some members of the local community informed or probably know
2 = Mother public about her lesbian identity (e.g., wears badges or holdshands with her partner in public)

Mother's discussion with child's school about her lesbian identity
0 = No
1 = Belief on mother's part that school staff know about her lesbian relationships but issue not discussed in any detail
2 = Discussions between mother and school staff about bringing children up in a lesbian family

Mother's feelings toward men
 1 = Negative
 2 = Indifferent
 3 = Positive
 4 = Emotional attachments with men
 5 = Sexual feelings toward men

Mother's involvement in lesbian politics prior to the original study
 0 = No political involvement
 1 = Political involvement but not public involvement
 2 = Occasional public political involvement
 3 = Frequent public political involvement

Mother's involvement in lesbian social groups
 0 = No involvement
 1 = Occasional attendance
 2 = Frequent attendance

Mother's preference for child's future sexual orientation
 0 = Prefers child to be heterosexual
 1 = No particular preference

Mother's rating of child's awareness of her lesbian identity
 0 = None
 1 = Some awareness
 2 = Fully aware

1991–1992 Follow-Up Interviews with Young Adults: Variables Used in the Statistical Analyses

FAMILY RELATIONSHIPS[1]

Mother's relationship style (since mother and father separated); interrater reliability ($r = .676$, $p = .004$)

1 = One exclusive cohabitation for the majority of the time
2 = Serial cohabiting relationships or one previous cohabiting relationship followed by noncohabiting relationships
3 = Serial noncohabiting relationships
4 = Nonexclusive relationships at some time after parental separation

Young adult's description of his/her relationship with mother currently; interrater reliability ($r = .733$, $p = .001$)

1 = Very negative (strong dislike and high levels of confrontation)
2 = Moderately negative
3 = Moderately positive
4 = Very positive (very enthusiastic description, nothing negative said except for isolated minor point)

Young adult's description of his/her relationship with father currently (if child no longer sees father but voices strong positive or negative feelings about him this is also rated); interrater reliability ($r = .871$, $p = .002$)

1 = Very negative (strong dislike and high levels of confrontation)
2 = Moderately negative

---

[1]Young people who reported that their mother had no new relationships after parental separation are excluded from variables referring to stepfamily relationships.

3 = Moderately positive
4 = Very positive (very enthusiastic description, nothing negative said except for isolated minor point)

Father's attitude toward mother's new relationships; interrater reliability (r = 1.000)
1 = Negative (father upset by mother's new relationships or opposed to them)
2 = Father appears not bothered by mother's new relationships or child does not know what father thinks of them (alternatively father has been positive about mother's relationships, although child senses some disapproval)
3 = Positive (father openly expresses support for mother's new relationship)

Child's description of his/her relationship with mother's main relationship partner; interrater reliability (r = .754, p = .001)
1 = Very negative (strong dislike and high levels of confrontation)
2 = Moderately negative
3 = Moderately positive
4 = Very positive (very enthusiastic description, nothing negative said except for isolated minor point)

Young adult's description of his/her relationship with mother's current relationship partner; interrater reliability (r = .819; p = .001)
1 = Very negative (strong dislike and high levels of confrontation)
2 = Moderately negative
3 = Moderately positive
4 = Very positive (very enthusiastic description, nothing negative said except for isolated minor point)

Involvement in child care by mother's main relationship partner; interrater reliability (r = .806, p < .001)
1 = Coparent (regarded as a second parent by child or as involved as mother in child care)
2 = Stepparent (less involved in child care than mother although some involvement of mother's partner in family activities)
3 = Mother's partner (minimal involvement with child, mother always involved in any activities partner and child do together)

Mother's happiness in her main relationship; interrater reliability (r = .858, p < .001)
1 = Relationship unhappy for a lot of the time
2 = Relationship happy at first but deteriorated
3 = Relationship unhappy initially but satisfaction improved
4 = Relationship happy (even if mother subsequently separated from her partner)

Conflict between mother and her main relationship partner; interrater reliability ($r = .775$, $p = .001$)
1 = Regular episodes of serious conflict during the relationship
2 = Frequent conflict only prior to the end of the relationship
3 = Interviewee remembers one or two serious conflicts
4 = No serious conflict remembered

Extent to which child felt emotionally burdened by mother's confidences; interrater reliability ($r = .930$, $p < .001$)
1 = Pleased that mother confided (nothing said to indicate any emotional burden)
2 = Mother never confided in child, or no evidence of any positive or negative feelings about receiving mother's confidences
3 = Mild emotional involvement (child sometimes felt upset or angry at receiving mother's confidence but at other times did not feel burdened)
4 = Heavy emotional burden, with child feeling emotionally involved in mother's problems (e.g., feeling upset or angry on mother's behalf), although child may not be fully aware of his/her own emotional involvement

Child's knowledge of mother's relationships; variable codes child's memories of how became aware of mother's relationships, not simply whether he/she mother had a male/female friend sharing the house; interrater reliability ($r = .704$, $p = .007$)
1 = Gradual awareness
2 = Particular incident
3 = Mother told
4 = No knowledge or not applicable

Mother's openness in showing physical intimacy in front of child; interrater reliability ($r = .782$, $p < .001$)
0 = Child feels comfortable with the level of physical intimacy seen
1 = Child feels uncomfortable about mother's physical intimacy with partner

Mother's involvement in feminist politics; interrater reliability ($r = .843$, $p < .001$)
0 = None
1 = Mother involved in feminist politics and/or child perceives mother to be a feminist

Mother's involvement in gay rights politics (lesbian mother group only); interrater reliability ($r = 1.000$)
0 = None
1 = Mother involved in gay and lesbian rights campaigns

Mother's attitude toward gays and lesbians (heterosexual mother group only); interrater reliability (r = .919, p = .014)
1 = Negative
2 = Don't know mother's attitude
3 = Tolerant or positive

Mother's attitude toward men; interrater reliability (r = 1.000)
0 = Mother is negative about men generally, either from a political feminist perspective or from anger toward or wariness of men in general
1 = Mother is positive about men generally (mother has gay or heterosexual male friends and does not criticize men in general)

Child's interpretation of mother's contentment with her identity; interrater reliability (r = .715, p = .004)
1 = Mother is negative about her identity and would have preferred to be both heterosexual and married.
2 = Mother has mixed feelings
3 = Mother is positive about her identity and has little problem with her identity either as a lesbian mother or as a nonmarried heterosexual mother

Feelings during adolescence about nontraditional family identity; interrater reliability (r = .804, p < .001)
1 = Resentful or opposed (either angry with mother because of her relationships or completely refused to acknowledge mother's identity even to self)
2 = Embarrassed (secretive about mother's relationship so that young person has either told no one or just one special person—but no evidence of any personal denial or resentment about mother's relationships)
3 = Accepting (pleased that mother is happy in her relationship; not upset by mother's identity; no attempt to keep the relationship secret from friends)
4 = Proud (very positive about mother's relationships and has made a public statement about mother's identity to a wider audience than just friends)

Young adult's current feelings about nontraditional family identity; interrater reliability (r = .866, p < .001)
1 = Resentful or opposed (either angry with mother because of her relationships or completely refuses to acknowledge mother's identity even to self)
2 = Embarrassed (secretive about mother's relationship so that young adult has either told no one or just one special person—but no evidence of any personal denial or resentment about mother's relationships)
3 = Accepting (pleased that mother is happy in her relationship; not

upset by mother's identity; no attempt to keep the relationship secret from friends)

4 = Proud (very positive about mother's relationships and has made a public statement about mother's identity to a wider audience than just friends)

PEER RELATIONSHIPS

Teased or bullied at school; interrater reliability ($r = 1.000$)

0 = Not teased
1 = Teased or bullied at least once during school days

Extent of teasing or bullying during school days; interrater reliability ($r = .940, p < .001$)

0 = Not teased
1 = Isolated incident
2 = More serious incidents of teasing prolonged over an academic year

Teased about mother's lifestyle or identity; interrater reliability ($r = 1.000$)

0 = Never teased about mother
1 = Teased about mother's lifestyle (either teased about mother being a lesbian or about mother having boyfriends or own illegitimacy)

Teased about own sexuality or gender-inappropriate behavior; interrater reliability ($r = .730, p = .002$)

0 = Never teased about sexuality or gender-inappropriateness
1 = Teased about own sexuality or gender-inappropriateness (e.g., called a sissy or a tomboy)

Whether and how the adolescent's friends knew about mother's relationships; interrater reliability ($r = .959, p < .001$)

1 = Friends didn't know
2 = Friends found out
3 = Friends probably knew, but it was never discussed
4 = Adolescent told at least one friend about mother having a relationship with her partner

Response of school friends to knowledge of mother's relationship; interrater reliability ($r = .843, p = .001$)

1 = Friends (or their parents) negative
2 = One friend negative at first but accepting of it to some extent by the time adolescent left school
3 = Friends accepting or never mentioned it
4 = Friends positive

Mother's openness about her lesbian identity in front of child's school friends (lesbian mother group only); interrater reliability (r = 1.000)

  0 = Young person felt that his/her mother was discreet enough
  1 = Young person felt uncomfortable because mother was too open about her lesbian identity (either in openly showing affection to her partner or through her appearance or through books, pictures, or objects around the house).

Mother's attitude toward young person bringing high school friends home; interrater reliability (r = .837, p < .001)

  1 = Young person feels that he/she had major difficulties bringing friends home even if mother or mother's partner was enthusiastic about friends
  2 = Young person had some difficulties about bringing friends home (either the young person was reluctant to bring friends home or mother/mother's partner was generally fine about friends but occasionally could be difficult)
  3 = Young person had no difficulties bringing friends home when mother or her partner was at home. Friends were always welcomed. Mother was positive about adolescent's friends.

Close gay or lesbian friend; interrater reliability (r = .675, p = .006)

  0 = No gay or lesbian friend, or interviewee now has much less contact with a friend who came out as gay or lesbian
  1 = Has known or has had a lesbian or gay friend (not including friends of parents)

Young adult's attitude toward gay and lesbian rights; interrater reliability (r = .829, p < .001)

  1 = Anti
  2 = Tolerant
  3 = Argued with friends for lesbian and gay rights and against prejudice
  4 = Publicly campaigned

Young adult's attitude toward women's rights; interrater reliability (r = .693, p = .009)

  0 = No interest in women's rights in society or antifeminist
  1 = Supports women's rights or self-defined feminist

INTIMATE RELATIONSHIPS

Prepubertal opposite-gender sexual experience; interrater reliability (r = .730, p = .002)

  0 = None or no memories
  1 = Memories of sexual contact before puberty with friends or siblings (e.g., kissing and holding hands, interest in seeing other child in the nude, genital touching)

Prepubertal same-gender sexual experience; interrater reliability (r = .849, p < .001)

0 = None or no memories

1 = Memories of sexual contact before puberty with friends or siblings (e.g., kissing and holding hands, interest in seeing other child in the nude, genital touching)

Curiosity or interest in same-gender sexual development during puberty; interrater reliability (r = .720, p = .003)

0 = None or avoidance of opportunities for this

1 = Curiosity or interest in physical development of others of same sex or some sexual or affectionate contact with them during puberty (e.g., sharing a bed or cuddling)

Same-gender sexual attraction; interrater reliability (r = 1.000)

0 = No same-gender attractions

1 = Some same-gender attraction (either at least one crush on a specific person or general nonspecific same gender attractions or sexual fantasies)

Same-gender sexual relationship; interrater reliability (r = 1.000)

0 = No same-gender sexual relationships

1 = At least one same-gender sexual relationship (minimum criteria for relationship defined as kissing)

Sexual identity; interrater reliability (r = 1.000)

0 = Heterosexual identity

1 = Gay/lesbian/bisexual identity or relationship commitment (interviewee has had more than one same-gender sexual relationship and wants to continue having same-gender relationships in the future)

Consideration of gay/lesbian relationship possibilities; interrater reliability (r = .948, p < .001)

1 = Might have gay/lesbian relationships in the future (or will continue to have gay/lesbian relationships in the future if already had one)

2 = Previously wondered about possibility of being gay/lesbian or thought about the possibility of having same-gender relationships, but thinks it is impossible that he/she will have them in the future

3 = Never thought that gay relationships were a possibility for him/her

Kinsey scale ratings of interviewee's crushes and sexual fantasies during adolescence (interrater reliability [r = .951, p < .001]); Kinsey scale ratings of interviewee's sexual relationships and sexual fantasies during adulthood (interrater reliability [r = .970, p < .001]); an abbreviated version of the Kinsey scale is given below:

0 = No physical contacts or psychic responses to the same sex; all sociosexual contacts and responses exclusively with the opposite gender

1 = Only incidental physical or psychic responses to same gender
2 = More than incidental same-gender experience and/or definite response to homosexual stimuli, although heterosexual experiences and/or reactions exceed homosexual ones
3 = Bisexual; equal heterosexual and homosexual experiences and reactions
4 = More same-gender than opposite-gender experience and psychic reactions, although some heterosexual activity and interest
5 = Almost exclusively homosexual experience and psychic reactions with only incidental heterosexual experience and responses
6 = Exclusively same-gender sociosexual contacts and responses

Young adult's cohabitation history (both same-gender and opposite-gender cohabitations included); interrater reliability ($r = .739, p = .001$)
1 = Never cohabited or married
2 = One current cohabitation or marital relationship
3 = One previous cohabitation or marital relationship (now finished)
4 = More than one cohabitation or marital relationship

Age at first cohabitation/marriage; interrater reliability ($r = 1.000$)

Number of months into relationship before cohabiting or marriage in first cohabitation/marital relationship; interrater reliability ($r = 1.000$)

Age at first heterosexual intercourse; interrater reliability ($r = 1.000$)

Number of sexual relationships (including same- and opposite-gender penetrative and nonpenetrative sexual relationships); interrater reliability ($r = .889, p < .001$)
0 = None
1 = 1 sexual relationship
2 = 2 to 4 sexual relationships
3 = 5 to 9 sexual relationships
4 = 10 to 14 sexual relationships
5 = Over 15 sexual relationships

Quality of current intimate relationship in terms of interviewee's expressed satisfaction with the relationship and the presence of possibly unresolvable problems within the relationship; interrater reliability ($r = .913, p = .001$)
1 = Major difficulties in the relationship that overshadow any satisfaction with the relationship (e.g., unresolved conflict or affairs); more hope that the difficulties will end rather than satisfaction that they are being dealt with
2 = Enjoyment of the relationship (although there are some problems that need to be overcome or lack of communication between relationship partners) but interviewee's general feeling is that these difficulties are being surmounted
3 = Clear enjoyment of the relationship, no lack of communication within the relationship, and no major problems

Level of conflict in interviewee's current intimate relationship; inter-rater reliability ($r = .883, p = .002$)

   1 = Serious disagreement in the preceding month

   2 = Serious disagreement in the previous 6 months either one or more major arguments or chronic low level conflict

   3 = Occasional irritability, but interviewee reports no serious disagreements in the preceding 6 months

Extent of communication between interviewee and his/her mother (or mother's partner) about adolescent sexual relationships (e.g., contraceptive needs or sexual orientation); interrater reliability ($r = .904, p < .001$)

   0 = Interviewee and mother/mother's partner never discussed sexual relationships during adolescence, although mother or mother's partner may have known about the interviewee's sexual relationships at that time

   1 = Mother or mother's partner talked to interviewee generally about contraception needs or sexual orientation but not in the context of a specific relationship

   2 = Interviewee and mother or mother's partner discussed contraception or sexual orientation as these issues arose within the context of a specific relationship

Whether interviewee is able to sleep with their relationship partner at mother's house with mother's knowledge; interrater reliability ($r = .967, p < .001$)

   0 = Mother or mother's partner refuse to let young person have relationship partner to sleep over, unless they are married

   1 = Interviewee is able to have nonmarital relationship partner sleep with him/her at mother's house only after interviewee has left home

   2 = Interviewee has permission to have relationship partner sleep with him/her at mother's house with mother's knowledge while interviewee is still living at home and unmarried

Mother's and/or mother's partner's general response to young person's relationship partners; interrater reliability ($r = .687, p = .007$)

   1 = Generally disapproving of interviewee's relationship partners

   2 = Mixed (mother/mother's partner may have disapproved of some relationship partners but approved of others, alternatively, interviewee may have felt that mother/mother's partner tolerated but did not welcome his/her partner

   3 = Positive (although the interviewee may have felt that his/her mother or her partner was being too welcoming to his/her partner)

Young adult's opinion of mother's preference for his/her sexual orientation (rated even if interviewee believed that mother had only a slight

preference for his/her future sexual orientation); interrater reliability
($r = .882, p < .001$)

   1 = Mother has preference for interviewee to have opposite-gender
       sexual relationships
   2 = Mother accepts either same-gender or opposite-gender sexual
       relationships (interviewee believes that mother has no prefer-
       ence, or interviewee has no idea what mother prefers)
   3 = Mother has preference for interviewee to have same-gender
       physical relationships

DEMOGRAPHIC VARIABLES
AND GENERAL WELL-BEING

Young person's age at time of follow-up interview

Educational qualifications achieved or expected to be achieved; interrater reliability ($r = 1.000$)

   1 = Left school at 16 with either no qualifications, some basic
       qualifications, or short work-related training course
   2 = Advanced educational qualifications or more substantial voca-
       tional qualification
   3 = Higher education degree (or interviewee has currently completed
       at least 1 year of a degree course)

Career history; interrater reliability ($r = .957, p < .001$)

   1 = Good career record (interviewee has never been dismissed be-
       cause of problems at work and has always been in employment)
   2 = Full-time student
   3 = Good career record currently, but some problems in getting
       started (either periods of unemployment or conflict at work lead-
       ing to job change or failure to complete a course of higher edu-
       cation that had been started)
   4 = Major problems currently, either currently in conflict at work
       or unemployed (because of conflicts in previous job or because
       of apathy) or in a recently begun special restart course after
       period of unemployment
   5 = Full-time child care responsibilities

Professional consultation for mental health problem (i.e., with medical doctor, psychiatrist, psychologist, counselor, or therapist); interrater reliability ($r = 1.000$)

   0 = Never requested professional help
   1 = Previously sought professional help for a health problem con-
       nected with anxiety, depression, suicide attempt, alcohol, drugs,
       or sleep difficulties

References

Acock, A. C., & Bengston, V. L. (1980). Socialization and attribution processes: Actual versus perceived similarity among parents and youth. *Journal of Marriage and the Family, 42,* 501–513.

Ahrons, C. R., & Wallisch, L. (1987). Parenting in the binuclear family: Relationships between biological and stepparents. In K. Pasley & M. Ihinger-Tallman (Eds.), *Remarriage and stepparenting: Current research and theory* (pp. 225–256). New York: Guilford Press.

Ainsworth, M. D. S. (1972). Attachment and dependency: A comparison. In J. L. Gewirtz (Ed.), *Attachment and dependency* (pp. 97–137). New York: Wiley.

Ainsworth, M. D. S. (1979). Attachment as related to mother–infant interaction. In J. Rosenblatt, R. A. Hinde, C. Beer, & M. Busnel (Eds.), *Advances in the study of behavior* (Vol. 9, pp. 1–51). Orlando, FL: Academic Press.

Ainsworth, M. D. S. (1982). Attachment: Retrospect and prospect. In C. M. Parkes & J. Stevenson-Hinde (Eds.), *The place of attachment in human behavior* (pp. 3–30). New York: Basic Books.

Ainsworth, M. D. S., Blehar, M., Waters, E., & Wall, S. (1978). *Patterns of attachment.* Hillsdale, NJ: Erlbaum.

Allen, I. (1987). *Education in sex and personal relationships.* London: Policy Studies Institute.

Allison, P. D., & Furstenberg, F. F. (1989). How marital dissolution affects children: Variations by age and sex. *Developmental Psychology, 25,* 540–549.

Amato, P. R., & Keith, B. (1991a). Parental divorce and the well-being of children: A meta-analysis. *Psychological Bulletin, 110,* 26–46.

Amato, P. R., & Keith, B. (1991b). Parental divorce and adult well-being: A meta-analysis. *Journal of Marriage and the Family, 53,* 43–58.

American Psychiatric Association. (1994). *Diagnostic and statistical manual of mental disorders* (4th ed.). Washington, DC: Author.

Arnup, K. (1995). Living in the margins: Lesbian families and the law. In K. Arnup (Ed.), *Lesbian parenting: Living with pride and prejudice* (pp. 378–398). Charlottetown, Canada: Gynergy.

Asher, S. R. (1990). Recent advances in the study of peer rejection. In S. R. Asher & J. D. Coie (Eds.), *Peer rejection in childhood* (pp. 3–14). New York: Cambridge University Press.

B v B. (1991). *Family Law, 21,* 174.

Bailey, J. M., & Pillard, R. C. (1991). A genetic study of male sexual orientation. *Archives of General Psychiatry, 48,* 1089–1096.

Bailey, J. M., Bobrow, D., Wolfe, M., & Mikach, S. (1995). Sexual orientation of adult sons of gay men. *Developmental Psychology, 31,* 124–129.

Bailey, J. M., Pillard, R. C., Neale, M. C., & Agyei, Y. (1993). Heritable factors influence sexual orientation in women. *Archives of General Psychiatry, 50,* 217–223.

Bandura, A. (1977). *Social learning theory.* Englewood Cliffs, NJ: Prentice-Hall.

Bandura, A. (1986). *Social foundations of thought and action: A social cognitive theory.* Englewood Cliffs, NJ: Prentice-Hall.

Bandura, A. (1989). Social cognitive theory. *Annals of Child Development, 6,* 1–60.

Baumrind, D. (1971). Current patterns of parental authority. *Developmental Psychology Monographs, 4*(Part 2), 1–103.

Beck, A., & Steer, R. (1987). *The Beck Depression Inventory manual.* San Antonio, TX: Psychological Corporation.

Bell, A. P., & Weinberg, M. S. (1978). *Homosexualities: A study of diversity among men and women.* New York: Simon & Schuster.

Bell, A. P., Weinberg, M. S., & Hammersmith, S. K. (1981). *Sexual preference: Its development in men and women.* Bloomington, IN: Indiana University Press.

Bene, E. (1965a). On the genesis of male homosexuality: An attempt at clarifying the role of the parents. *British Journal of Psychiatry, 111,* 803–813.

Bene, E. (1965b). On the genesis of female homosexuality. *British Journal of Psychiatry, 111,* 815–821.

Berg, D. H. (1985). Reality construction at the family/society interface: The internalization of family themes and values. *Adolescence, 20*(79), 605–618.

Bieber, I., Dain, H., Dince, P., Drellick, M., Grand, H., Gondlack, R., Kremer, R., Rifkin, A., Wilber, C., & Bieber, T. (1962). *Homosexuality: A psychoanalytic study.* New York: Basic Books.

Biller, H. B. (1974). *Paternal deprivation.* Lexington, MA: Heath.

Blumstein, P., & Schwartz, P. (1983). *American couples: Money, work, and sex.* New York: Morrow.

Bowlby, J. (1969). *Attachment and loss: Vol. 1. Attachment.* London: Hogarth Press.

Bowlby, J. (1973). *Attachment and loss: Vol. 2. Separation: Anxiety and anger*. London: Hogarth Press.

Bowlby, J. (1980). *Attachment and Loss: Vol. 3. Loss*. London: Hogarth Press.

Bozett, F. W. (1987). Children of gay fathers. In F. W. Bozett (Ed), *Gay and lesbian parents* (pp. 39–57). London: Praeger.

Bozett, F. W. (1988). Social control of identity by children of gay fathers. *Western Journal of Nursing Research, 10*, 550–565.

Brand, E., Clingempeel, G., & Bowen-Woodward, K. (1988). Family relationships and children's psychological adjustment in stepmother and stepfather families. In E. M. Hetherington & J. D. Arasteh (Eds.), *Impact of divorce, single parenting and stepparenting on children* (pp. 299–324). Hillsdale, NJ: Erlbaum.

Breakwell, G. M., & Fife-Schaw, C. (1992). Sexual activities and preferences in a United Kingdom sample of 16- to 20-year-olds. *Archives of Sexual Behavior, 21*, 271–293.

Bromam, S. H., Nichols, P. L., & Kennedy, W. A. (1975). *Pre-school IQ: Parental and early development correlates*. Hillsdale, NJ: Erlbaum.

Brophy, J. (1989). Custody law, child care and inequality in Britain. In C. Smart & S. Sevenhuijsen (Eds.), *Child custody and the politics of gender* (pp. 217–242). London: Routledge.

Brophy, J. (1992). New families, judicial decision-making, and children's welfare. *Canadian Journal of Women and the Law, 5*, 484–497.

Brown, G. W., & Rutter, M. L. (1966). The measurement of family activities and relationships: A methodological study. *Human Relations, 19*, 241–263.

Burns, A. (1992). *Mother-headed families: An international perspective and the case of Australia* (Social Policy Report, 4. No. 124). Melbourne, Australia: Australian Institute of Family Studies.

Bussey, K., & Bandura, A. (1984). Influence of gender constancy and social power on sex-linked modeling. *Journal of Personality and Social Psychology, 47*, 1292–1302.

Byne, W., & Parsons, B. (1993). Human sexual orientation: The biologic theories reappraised. *Archives of General Psychiatry, 50*, 228–239.

Carter, D. B. (1987). The roles of peers in sex role socialization. In D. B. Carter (Ed.), *Current conceptions of sex roles and stereotyping* (pp. 101–121). New York: Praeger.

Cartledge, S., & Ryan, J. (1983). *Sex and love: New thoughts on old contradictions*. London: Women's Press.

Cassidy, J. (1988). Child–mother attachment and the self in six-year-olds. *Child Development, 59*, 121–134.

Cherlin, A., Furstenberg, F., Chase-Lansdale, P., Kiernan, K. E., Robins, P. K., Morrison, D. R., & Teitler, J. O. (1991). Longitudinal studies of effects of divorce on children in Great Britain and the United States. *Science, 252*, 1386–1389.

Clingempeel, W. G., & Segal, S. (1986). Stepparent–stepchild relationships and the psychological adjustment of children in stepmother and stepfather families. *Child Development, 57,* 474–484.

Cockett, M., & Tripp, J. (1994). *The Exeter Family Study: Family breakdown and its impact on children.* Exeter, UK: University of Exeter Press.

Coie, J. D., & Cillessen, H. N. (1993). Peer rejection: Origins and effects on children's development. *Current Directions in Psychological Science, 2,* 89–92.

Cox, A., & Rutter, M. (1985). Diagnostic appraisal and interviewing. In M. Rutter & L. Hersov (Eds.), *Child and adolescent psychiatry* (2nd Ed., pp. 233–248). Oxford, UK: Blackwell.

Crockenberg, S. (1981). Infant irritability, mother responsiveness, and social support influences on the security of infant–mother attachment. *Child Development, 52,* 857–65.

Deevey, S. (1989). When mom or dad comes out: Helping adolescents cope with homophobia. *Journal of Psychosocial Nursing and Mental Health Services, 27,* 33–36.

Diamond, M. (1993). Homosexuality and bisexuality in different populations. *Archives of Sexual Behavior, 22,* 291–310.

Dittman, R. W., Kappes, M. E., & Kappes, M. H. (1992). Sexual behavior in adolescent and adult females with congenital adrenal hyperplasia. *Psychoneuroendocrinology, 17,* 1–18.

Dunn, J., & McGuire, S. (1992). Sibling and peer relationships in childhood. *Journal of Child Psychology and Psychiatry, 33,* 67–105.

Dunne, G. D. (1992). *Sexuality, home-life and the structuring of employment.* Unpublished doctoral dissertation, University of Cambridge, Cambridge, UK.

Editors of the Harvard Law Review. (1990). *Sexual orientation and the law.* Cambridge, MA: Harvard University Press.

Ehrhardt, A. A., Meyer-Bahlburg, H. F. L., Rosen, L., Feldman, L., Veridiano, N., Zimmerman, I., & McEwen, B. (1985). Sexual orientation after prenatal exposure to exogenous estrogen. *Archives of Sexual Behavior, 14,* 57–77.

Elliott, J., Ochiltree, G., Richards, M., Sinclair, C., & Tasker, F. (1990). Divorce and children: A British challenge to the Wallerstein view. *Family Law, 20,* 309–310.

Elliott, B. J., & Richards, M. P. M. (1991). Children of divorce: Educational performance, and behaviour, before and after parental separation. *International Journal of Law and the Family, 5,* 258–276.

Emery, R. E. (1982). Interparental conflict and the children of discord and divorce. *Psychological Bulletin, 92,* 310–330.

Emery, R. E. (1988). *Marriage, divorce and children's adjustment.* London: Sage.

Ettore, E. M. (1980). *Lesbians, women and society.* London: Routledge.

Evans, R. (1969). Childhood parental relationships of homosexual men. *Journal of Consulting and Clinical Psychology, 33,* 129–135.

Fagot, B. I., & Hagan, R. (1991). Observations of parent reactions to sex-stereotyped behaviors, *Child Development, 62,* 617–628.

Falk, P. J. (1989). Lesbian mothers: Psychosocial assumptions in family law. *American Psychologist, 44,* 941–947.

Ferri, E. (1976). Growing up in a one-parent family. Windsor, UK: National Foundation for Education Research.

Fine, R. (1987). Psychoanalytic theory. In L. Diamant (Ed.), *Male and female homosexuality: Psychological approaches* (pp. 81–95). London: Hemisphere.

Finkelhor, D., & Russell, D. (1984). Women as perpetrators: Review of the evidence. In D. Finkelhor (Ed.), *Child sexual abuse: New theory and research* (pp. 171–187). New York: Free Press.

Flaks, D. K., Ficher, I., Masterpasqua, F., & Joseph, G. (1995). Lesbians choosing motherhood: A comparative study of lesbian and heterosexual parents and their children. *Developmental Psychology, 31,* 105–114.

Flewelling, R. L., & Bauman, K. E. (1990). Family structure as a predictor of initial substance use and sexual intercourse in early adolescence. *Journal of Marriage and the Family, 52,* 171–181.

Frank, E., Prien, R. F., Jarrett, R. B., Keller, M. B., Kupfer, D. J., Lavori, P. W., Rush, A. J., & Weissman, M. M. (1991). Conceptualization and rationale for consensus definitions of terms in major depressive disorder. *Archives of General Psychiatry, 48,* 851–858.

Freud, S. (1953). Three essays on the theory of sexuality. In J. Strachey (Ed. and Trans.), *The standard edition of the complete psychological works of Sigmund Freud* (Vol. 7, pp. 125–263). London: Hogarth Press. (Original work published 1905)

Freud, S. (1955). Beyond the pleasure principle. In J. Strachey (Ed. and Trans.), *The standard edition of the complete psychological works of Sigmund Freud* (Vol. 18, pp. 3–68). London: Hogarth Press. (Original work published 1920)

Freud, S. (1964). New introductory lectures on psycho-analysis (Lecture XXXIII: Femininity). In J. Strachey (Ed. and Trans.), *The standard edition of the complete psychological works of Sigmund Freud* (Vol. 22, pp. 112–135). London: Hogarth Press. (Original work published 1933)

Friedman, R. C. (1988). *Male homosexuality: A contemporary psychoanalytic perspective.* New Haven, CT: Yale University Press.

Furstenberg, F. F. (1987). The new extended family: The experience of parents and children after remarriage. In K. Pasley & M. Ihinger-Tallman (Eds.), *Remarriage and stepparenting: Current research and theory* (pp. 42–61). New York: Guilford Press.

Gagnon, J. H. (1977). *Human sexuality.* Glenview IL: Scott, Foresman.

Gagnon, J. H. (1990). Gender preference in erotic relations: The Kinsey scale and sexual scripts. In D. P. McWhirter, S. A. Sanders, & J. M. Reinisch (Eds.), *Homosexuality/heterosexuality: Concepts of sexual orientation* (pp. 177–207). Oxford, UK: Oxford University Press.

Gagnon, J. H., & Simon, W. S. (1973). *Sexual conduct: The social sources of human sexuality*. Chicago: Aldine Books.

Glenn, N. D., & Kramer, K. K. (1985). The psychological well-being of adult children of divorce. *Journal of Marriage and the Family, 47*, 905–991.

Glenn, N. D., & Kramer, K. K. (1987). The marriages and divorces of the children of divorce. *Journal of Marriage and the Family, 49*, 811–825.

Goffman, E. (1963). *Stigma: Notes on the management of a spoiled identity*. London: Penguin.

Goldberg, D., & Huxley, P. (1992). *Common mental disorders: A biosocial model*. London: Routledge.

Golden, C. (1994). Our politics and choices: The feminist movement and sexual orientation. In B. Greene & G. M. Herek (Eds.), *Lesbian and gay psychology: Theory, research and clinical applications* (pp. 54–70). Beverly Hills, CA: Sage.

Golombok, S., Tasker, F., & Murray, C. (in press). Children raised in fatherless families from infancy: Family relationships and the socioemotional development of children of lesbian and single heterosexual mothers. *Journal of Child Psychology and Psychiatry*.

Golombok, S., Spencer, A., & Rutter, M. (1983). Children in lesbian and single-parent households: Psychosexual and psychiatric appraisal. *Journal of Child Psychology and Psychiatry, 24*, 551–572.

Golombok, S., & Tasker, F. (1994). Children in lesbian and gay families: Theories and evidence. *Annual Review of Sex Research, 5*, 73–100.

Golombok, S., & Tasker, F. (1996). Do parents influence the sexual orientation of their children? Findings from a longitudinal study of lesbian families. *Developmental Psychology, 32*, 3–11.

Gonsiorek, J. C., & Weinrich, J. D. (1991). The definition and scope of sexual orientation. In J. C. Gonsiorek, & J. D. Weinrich (Eds.), *Homosexuality: Research implications for public policy* (pp. 1–12). London: Sage.

Gottman, J. S. (1990). Children of gay and lesbian parents. In F. W. Bozett & M. B. Sussman (Eds.), *Homosexuality and Family Relations* (pp. 177–196). New York: Harrington Park.

Goy, R. W., & McEwen, B. S. (1980). *Sexual differentiation in the brain*. Cambridge, MA: MIT Press.

Graham, P., & Rutter, M. (1968). The reliability and validity of the psychiatric assessment of the child: II. Interview with the parent. *British Journal of Psychiatry, 114*, 581–592.

Green, R. (1987). *The "sissy boy syndrome" and the development of homosexuality.* New Haven, CT: Yale University Press.

Green, R. (1992). *Sexual science and the law.* Cambridge, MA: Harvard University Press.

Green, R., Mandel, J. B., Hotvedt, M. E., Gray, J., & Smith, L. (1986). Lesbian mothers and their children: A comparison with solo parent heterosexual mothers and their children. *Archives of Sexual Behavior, 15,* 167–184.

Green, R., Williams, K., & Goodman, M. (1982). Ninety-nine "tomboys" and "non-tomboys": Behavioral contrasts and demographic similarities. *Archives of Sexual Behavior, 11,* 247–266.

Grossmann, K. E., Grossmann, K., Spangler, G., Suess, G., & Unzer, L. (1985). Maternal sensitivity in northern Germany. In I. Bretherton & E. Waters (Eds.), Growing points of attachment theory and research. *Monographs of the Society for Research in Child Development, 50*(Serial No. 209; 1–2), 233–256.

Hall, M. (1978). Lesbian families: Cultural and clinical issues. *Social Work, 23,* 380–385.

Hamer, D., Hu, S., Magnuson, V., Hu, N., & Pattatucci, A. (1993). A linkage between DNA markers on the X chromosome and male sexual orientation. *Science, 261,* 321–327.

Hart, J. (1981). Theoretical explanations in practice. In J. Hart & D. Richardson (Eds.), *The theory and practice of homosexuality* (pp. 38–67). London: Routledge.

Henecken, J. D. (1984). Conceptualizations of homosexual behavior which preclude homosexual self-labeling. *Journal of Homosexuality, 9,* 53–63.

Hernandez, D. J. (1988). Demographic trends and the living arrangements of children. In E. M. Hetherington & J. D. Arasteh (Eds.), *The impact of divorce, single parenting and stepparenting on children* (pp. 3–22). Hillsdale, NJ: Erlbaum.

Herzog, E., & Sudia, C. E. (1973). Children in fatherless families. In B. M. Campbell & H. N. Ricciuti (Eds.), *Review of child development research* (pp. 161–231). Chicago: University of Chicago Press.

Hess, R. D., & Camara, K. A. (1979). Post-divorce relationships as mediating factors in the consequences of divorce for children. *Journal of Social Issues, 35,* 79–96.

Hetherington, E. M. (1988). Parents, children and siblings six years after divorce. In R. Hinde & J. Stevenson-Hinde (Eds.), *Relationships within families* (pp. 311–331). Cambridge, UK: Cambridge University Press.

Hetherington, E. M. (1989). Coping with family transitions: Winners, losers, and survivors. *Child Development, 60,* 1–14.

Hetherington, E. M., & Camara, K. A. (1988). The effects of family dissolution and reconstitution on children. In N. D. Glenn & M.

T. Coleman (Eds.), *Family relations: A reader* (pp. 420–431). Chicago: Dorsey Press.

Hetherington, E. M., & Clingempeel, W. G. (1992). Coping with marital transitions. *Monographs of the Society for Research in Child Development, 57,* (Nos. 2–3).

Hetherington, E. M., Cox, M., & Cox, R. (1982). Effects of divorce on parents and children. In M. E. Lamb (Ed.), *Nontraditional families: Parenting and child development* (pp. 233–288). Hillsdale, NJ: Erlbaum.

Hetherington, E. M., Cox, M., & Cox, R. (1985). Long-term effects of divorce and remarriage on the adjustment of children. *Journal of the American Academy of Psychology, 24,* 518–530.

Hines, M., & Green, R. (1990). Human hormonal and neural correlates of sex-typed behaviors. *Review of Psychiatry, 10,* 536–555.

Hitchins, D. J., & Kirkpatrick, M. (1986). Lesbian mothers/gay fathers. In E. Benedek & D. Shetsky (Eds.), *Emerging issues in child psychiatry and the law* (Vol. II, pp. 115–126). New York: Brunner/Mazel.

Hoeffer, B. (1981). Children's acquisition of sex-role behavior in lesbian-mother families. *American Journal of Orthopsychiatry, 5,* 536–544.

Huggins, S. L. (1989). A comparative study of self-esteem of adolescent children of divorced lesbian mothers and divorced heterosexual mothers. In F. Bozett (Ed.), *Homosexuality and the family* (pp. 123–135). New York: Harrington Park.

Huston, A. (1983). Sex typing. In E. M. Hetherington (Ed.), *Handbook of child psychology: Vol. 4. Socialization, personality and social development* (pp. 387–467). New York: Wiley.

Isabella, R. A., & Belsky, J. (1991). Interactional synchrony and the origins of infant–mother attachment: A replication study. *Child Development, 62,* 373–384.

Isabella, R. A., Belsky, J., & von Eye, A. (1989). Origins of infant–mother attachment: An examination of interactional synchrony during the infant's first year. *Developmental Psychology, 25,* 12–21.

Izard, C. E., Haynes, M., Chisholm, G., & Baak, K. (1991). Emotional determinants of infant–mother attachment. *Child Development, 62,* 906–917.

Javaid, G. A. (1983). The sexual development of the adolescent daughter of a homosexual mother. *Journal of the American Academy of Child Psychiatry, 22,* 196–201.

Johnson, A. M., & Wadsworth, J. (1994). Heterosexual partnerships. In A. M. Johnson, J. Wadsworth, K. Wellings, & J. Field (Eds.), *Sexual attitudes and lifestyles* (pp. 110–144). Oxford, UK: Blackwell Scientific.

Kalter, N. (1977). Children of divorce in an outpatient population. *American Journal of Orthopsychiatry, 47,* 40–51.

Kalter, N., Riemer, B., Brickman, A., & Chen, J. W. (1985). Implications of divorce for female development. *Journal of the American Academy of Child Psychiatry, 24,* 538–544.

Kaye, H., Berl, S., Clare, J., Eleston, M., Gershwin, B., Gershwin, P., Kogan, L., Torda, C., & Wilbur, C. (1967). Homosexuality in women. *Archives of General Psychiatry, 17,* 626–634.

Kiernan, K. E. (1992). The impact of family disruption in childhood on transitions made in young adult life. *Population Studies, 46,* 213–234.

Kinsey, A. C., Pomeroy, W. B., & Martin, C. E. (1948). *Sexual behavior in the human male.* Philadelphia: Saunders.

Kinsey, A. C., Pomeroy, W. B., & Martin, C. E. (1953) *Sexual behavior in the human female.* Philadelphia: Saunders.

Kirkpatrick, M. (1987). Clinical implications of lesbian mother studies. *Journal of Homosexuality, 13,* 201–211.

Kirkpatrick, M., Smith, C., & Roy, R. (1981). Lesbian mothers and their children: A comparative survey. *American Journal of Orthopsychiatry, 51,* 545–551.

Kitzinger, C. (1987). *The social construction of lesbianism.* London: Sage.

Kitzinger, C. (1995). Social constructionism: Implications for lesbian and gay psychology. In A. R. D'Augelli & C. J. Patterson (Eds.), *Lesbian, gay and bisexual identities over the lifespan: Psychological perspectives* (pp. 136–161). Oxford, UK: Oxford University Press.

Kitzinger, C., & Coyle, A. (1995). Lesbian and gay couples: Speaking of difference. *The Psychologist, 8,* 64–69.

Kitzinger, C., & Wilkinson, S. (1995). Transitions from heterosexuality to lesbianism: The discursive production of lesbian identities. *Developmental Psychology, 31,* 95–104.

Kitzinger, C., Wilkinson, S., & Perkins, R. (1992). Theorizing heterosexuality. *Feminism and Psychology, 2,* 293–324.

Klagsbrun, M., & Bowlby, J. (1976). Responses to separation from parents: A clinical test for young children. *British Journal of Projective Psychology, 21,* 7–21.

Kleber, D. J., Howell, R. J., & Tibbits-Kleber, A. L. (1986). The impact of parental homosexuality in child custody cases: A review of the literature. *Bulletin of the American Academy of Psychiatry and Law, 14,* 81–87.

Knox, E. G., MacArthur, C., & Simons, K. J. (1993). *Sexual behaviour and AIDS in Britain.* London: Her Majesty's Stationery Office.

Kohlberg, L. (1966). A cognitive-developmental analysis of children's sex-role concepts and attitudes. In E. E. Maccoby (Ed.), *The development of sex differences* (pp. 82–173). Stanford, CA: Stanford University Press.

Kuh, D., & Maclean, M. (1990). Women's childhood experience of parental separation and their subsequent health and socioeconomic status in adulthood. *Journal of Biosocial Science, 22,* 121–135.

Kupersmidt, J. B., Coie, J. D., & Dodge, K. A. (1990). The role of poor peer relationships in the development of disorder. In S. R. Asher & J. D. Coie (Eds.), *Peer rejection in childhood* (pp. 274–305). Cambridge, UK: Cambridge University Press.

Lamborn, S., Mounts, N., Steinberg, L., & Dornbusch, S. (1991). Patterns of competence and adjustment among adolescents from authoritative, authoritarian, indulgent and neglectful homes. *Child Development, 62,* 1049–1065.

Langlois, J. H., & Downs, A. C. (1980). Mothers, fathers and peers as socialization agents of sex-typed play behaviors in young children. *Child Development, 51,* 1237–1247.

Lesbian Mothers Group. (1989). "A word might slip and that would be it." Lesbian mothers and their children. In L. Holly (Ed.), *Girls and sexuality: Teaching and learning* (pp. 122–129). Milton Keynes, UK: Open University Press.

LeVay, S. (1991). A difference in hypothalamic structure between heterosexual and homosexual men. *Science, 253,* 1034–1037.

Lewis, K. G. (1980). Children of lesbians: Their point of view. *Social Work, 25,* 198–203.

Lewis, M., Feiring, C., McGuffog, C., & Jaskir, J. (1984). Predicting psycho-pathology in six-year-olds from early social relations. *Child Development, 55,* 123–136.

Londerville, S., & Main, M. (1981). Security of attachment, compliance, and maternal training methods in the second year of life. *Developmental Psychology, 17,* 289–299.

Lutkenhaus, P., Grossmann, K. E., & Grossmann, K. (1985). Infant–mother attachment at twelve months and style of interaction with a stranger at the age of three years. *Child Development, 56,* 1538–1542.

Lytton, H., & Romney, D. M. (1991). Parents' differential socialization of boys and girls: A meta-analysis. *Psychological Bulletin, 109,* 267–296.

Maccoby, E. E. (1988). Gender as a social category. *Developmental Psychology, 45,* 513–520.

Maccoby, E. E. (1990). Gender and relationships: A developmental account. *American Psychologist, 45,* 513–520.

Maccoby, E. E., & Jacklin, C. N. (1974). *The psychology of sex differences.* Stanford, CA: Stanford University Press.

Maccoby, E. E., & Martin, J. A. (1983). Socialization in the context of the family: Parent–child interaction. In E.M. Hetherington (Ed.), P. H. Mussen (Series Ed.), *Handbook of child psychology: Vol 4. Socialization, personality, and social development* (pp. 1–101). New York: Wiley.

Maclean, M. (1991). *Surviving divorce: Women's resources after separation.* New York: Macmillan.

Maclean, M., & Wadsworth, M. E. J. (1988). The interests of children after parental divorce: A long-term perspective. *International Journal of Law and the Family, 2,* 155–166.

Main, M., Kaplan, N., & Cassidy, J. (1985). Security in infancy, childhood and adulthood: A move to the level of representation. In I. Bretherton & E. Waters (Eds.), Growing points in attachment theory and research. *Monographs of the Society for Research in Child Development, 50*(Serial No. 209; 1–2), 66–104.

Martin, A. (1993). *The lesbian and gay parenting handbook.* New York: HarperCollins.

Martin, C. L. (1989, April). *Beyond knowledge-based conceptions of schematic processing.* Paper presented at the Society for Reserach in Child Development, Kansas City, KS.

Martin, C. L. (1991). The role of cognition in understanding gender effects. In H. Reese (Ed.) *Advances in child development and behavior* (Vol. 23, pp. 113–164). New York: Academic Press.

Martin, C. L. (1993). New directions for assessing children's gender knowledge. *Developmental Review, 13,* 184–204.

Martin, C. L., & Halverson, C. (1981). A schematic processing model of sex typing and stereotyping in children. *Child Development, 52,* 1119–1134.

Matas, L., Arend, R. A., & Sroufe, L. A. (1978). Continuity of adaptation in the second year: The relationship between quality of attachment and later competence. *Child Development, 49,* 547–556.

McCandlish, B. (1987). Against all odds: Lesbian mother family dynamics. In F. W. Bozett (Ed.), *Gay and lesbian parents* (pp. 23–26). New York: Praeger.

Meikle, S., Peitchinis, J. A., & Pearce, K. (1985). *Teenage sexuality.* London: Taylor & Francis.

Meyer-Bahlburg, H. F. L. (1984). Psychoendocrine research on sexual orientation: Current status and future options. *Progress in Brain Research, 61,* 375–398.

Meyer-Bahlburg, H. F. L., Ehrhardt, A. A., Rosen, L. R., Gruen, R. S., Veridiano, N. P., Vann, F. H., & Neuwalder, H. F. (1995). Prenatal estrogens and the development of homosexual orientation. *Developmental Psychology, 31,* 12–21.

Miller, B. (1979). Gay fathers and their children. *Family coordinator, 28,* 544–552.

Miller, J. A., Jacobsen, R. B., & Bigner, J. J. (1981). The child's home environment for lesbian vs. heterosexual mothers: A neglected area of research. *Journal of Homosexuality, 7,* 49–56.

Minuchin, S. (1974). *Families and family therapy.* London: Tavistock.

Mischel, W. (1966). A social learning view of sex differences in behavior. In E. E. Maccoby (Ed.), *The development of sex differences* (pp. 56–81). Stanford, CA: Stanford University Press.

Mischel, W. (1970). Sex-typing and socialization. In P. Mussen (Ed.),

Carmichael's manual of child psychology (Vol. 2, pp. 3–72). New York: Wiley.

Money, J. (1987). Sin, sickness or status? Homosexual gender identity and psychoneuroendocrinology. *American Psychologist, 42,* 384–399.

Money, J. (1988). *Gay, straight or in-between: The sexology of erotic orientation.* New York: Oxford University Press.

Money, J., Schwartz, M., & Lewis, V. (1984). Adult erotosexual status and fetal hormonal masculinization and demasculinization: 46, XX congenital virilizing adrenal hyperplasia and 46, XY androgen-insensitivity syndrome compared. *Psychoneuroendocrinology, 9,* 405–414.

Moore, D. S., & Erickson, P. I. (1985). Age, gender and ethnic differences in sexual contraceptive knowledge, attitudes, and behavior. *Family and Community Health, 8,* 38–51.

Mucklow, B. M., & Phelan, G. K. (1979). Lesbian and traditional mothers' responses to child behavior and self-concept. *Psychological Reports, 44,* 880–882.

Newcombe, M. (1985). The role of perceived relative parent personality in the development of heterosexuals, homosexuals and transvestites. *Archives of Sexual Behavior, 14,* 147–164.

Noller, P., & Callan, V. (1991). *The adolescent in the family.* London: Routledge.

Pagelow, M. D. (1980). Heterosexual and lesbian single mothers: A comparison of problems, coping and solutions. *Journal of Homosexuality, 5,* 198–204.

Parker, J. G., & Asher, S. R. (1987). Peer relations and later personal adjustment: Are low-accepted children at risk? *Psychological Bulletin, 102,* 357–389.

Pasley, K., & Ihinger-Tallman, M. (1987). The evolution of a field of investigation: Issues and concerns. In K. Pasley & M. Ihinger-Tallman (Eds.), *Remarriage and stepparenting: Current research and theory* (pp. 303–313). New York: Guilford Press.

Pastor, D. L. (1981). The quality of mother–infant attachment and its relationship to toddlers' initial sociability with peers. *Developmental Psychology, 17,* 326–335.

Patterson, C. J. (1992). Children of lesbian and gay parents. *Child Development, 63,* 1025–1042.

Patterson, C. J. (1994). Children of the lesbian baby boom: Behavioral adjustment, self-concepts, and sex-role identity. In B. Greene & G. M. Herek (Eds.), *Contemporary perspectives on lesbian and gay psychology: Theory, research and application* (pp. 156–175). Beverly Hills, CA: Sage.

Patterson, C. J. (1995a). Lesbian mothers, gay fathers, and their children. In A. R. D'Augelli & C. J. Patterson (Eds.), *Lesbian, gay and bisexual identities over the lifespan: Psychological perspectives* (pp. 262–290). Oxford, UK: Oxford University Press.

Patterson, C. J. (1995b). Families of the lesbian baby boom: Parents' division of labor and children's adjustment. *Developmental Psychology, 31,* 115–123.

Paul, J. P. (1986). *Growing up with a gay, lesbian, or bisexual parent: An exploratory study of experiences and perceptions.* Unpublished doctoral dissertation, University of California at Berkeley.

Pederson, D., Moran, G., Sitko, C., Campbell, K., Ghesquire, K., & Acton, H. (1990). Maternal sensitivity and the security of infant–mother attachment: A Q-sort study. *Child Development, 61,* 1974–1983.

Pennington, S. B. (1987). Children of lesbian mothers. In F. W. Bozett (Ed.), *Gay and lesbian parents* (pp. 58–74). New York: Praeger.

Perry, D. G., & Bussey, K. (1979). The social learning theory of sex difference: Imitation is alive and well. *Journal of Personality and Social Psychology, 37,* 1699–1712.

Plummer, K. (1975). *Sexual stigma: An interactionist account.* London: Routledge.

Polikoff, N. (1990). This child does have two mothers: Redefining parenthood to meet the needs of children in lesbian-mother and other nontraditional families. *Georgetown Law Journal, 78,* 459–575.

Pope, H., & Mueller, C. W. (1976). The intergenerational transmission of marital instability: Comparisons by sex and race. *Journal of Social Issues, 32,* 49–66.

Puryear, D. (1983). *A comparison between the children of lesbian mothers and the children of heterosexual mothers.* Unpublished doctoral dissertation, California School of Professional Psychology, Berkeley.

Quinton, D., & Rutter, M. (1988). *Parenting Breakdown: The making and breaking of intergenerational links.* Aldershot, UK: Avebury Gower.

Quinton, D., Rutter, M., & Rowlands, O. (1976). An evaluation of an interview assessment of marriage. *Psychological Medicine, 6,* 577–586.

Rafkin, L. (Ed.). (1990). *Different mothers: Sons and daughters of lesbians talk about their lives.* Pittsburgh: Cleis.

Rand, C., Graham, D. L. R., & Rawlings, E. I. (1982). Psychological health and factors the court seeks to control in lesbian mother custody trials. *Journal of Homosexuality, 8,* 27–39.

Richardson, D. (1981). Theoretical perspectives on homosexuality. In J. Hart & D. Richardson (Eds.), *The theory and practice of homosexuality* (pp. 5–37). London: Routledge.

Richardson, D. (1983). The dilemma of essentiality in homosexual theory. *Journal of Homosexuality, 9,* 79–90.

Ricketts, W., & Achtenberg, R. (1990). Adoption and foster parenting for lesbians and gay men: Creating new traditions in family. In F. W. Bozett & M. B. Sussman (Eds.), *Homosexuality and family relations* (pp. 83–118). New York: Praeger.

Riddle, D. I. (1978). Relating to children: Gays as role models. *Journal of Social Issues, 34,* 38–58.

Rivera, R. R. (1991). Sexual orientation and the law. In J. C. Gonsiorek & L. D. Weinrich (Eds.), *Homosexuality: Research implications for public policy* (pp. 81–100). Newbury Park, CA, Sage.

Roberts, C. W., Green, R., Williams, K., & Goodman, M. (1987). Boyhood gender identity development: A statistical contrast of two family groups. *Developmental Psychology, 23,* 544–557.

Roll, J. (1992). *Lone parent families in the European community.* London: European Family and Social Policy Unit.

Rose, J. (1990). Hanna Segal interview. *Women: A Cultural Review, 1,* 198–214.

Rust, J., Bennun, I., Crowe, M., & Golombok, S. (1988). *The handbook of the Golombok–Rust Inventory of Marital State.* Windsor, UK: NFER-Nelson.

Rutter, M. (1971). Parent–child separation: Psychological effects on children. *Journal of Child Psychology and Psychiatry, 12,* 233–260.

Rutter, M., & Brown, G. W. (1966). The reliability and validity of measures of family life and relationships in families containing a psychiatric patient. *Social Psychiatry, 1,* 38–53.

Rutter, M., Cox, A., Tupling, C., Berger, M., & Yule, W. (1975). Attainment and adjustment in two geographical areas: The prevalence of psychiatric disorder. *British Journal of Psychiatry, 126,* 493–541.

Rutter, M., & Madge, N. (1976). *Cycles of disadvantage: A review of research.* London: Heinemann.

Rutter, M., Quinton, D., & Hill, J. (1990). Adult outcome of institution-reared children: Male and females compared. In L. Robins & M. Rutter (Eds), *Straight and devious pathways from childhood to adulthood* (pp. 135–157). Cambridge, UK: Cambridge University Press.

Rutter, M., Tizard, J., & Whitmore, K. (1970). *Education, health and behaviour.* London: Longmans.

Safer, J., & Reiss, B. (1975). Two approaches to the study of female homosexuality: A critical and comparative review. *International Mental Health Newsletter, 17,* 11–13.

Saffron, L. (1994). *Challenging conceptions.* London: Cassell.

Saghir, M. T., & Robins, E. (1973). *Male and female homosexuality: A comprehensive investigation.* Baltimore: Williams & Wilkins.

Sandfort, T., van Zessen, G., & de Vroome, E. (1994, June 28–July 2). *Kinsey's zeros and ones: Do they really differ?* Paper presented at the 20th Annual Meeting of the International Academy of Sex Research, Edinburgh, Scotland.

Siegelman, M. (1974). Parental background of male homosexuals and heterosexuals. *Archives of Sexual Behaviour, 6,* 89–96.

Sigelman, C. K., Howell, J. L., Cornell, D. P., Cutright, J. D., & Dewey, J. C. (1991). Courtesy stigma: The social implications of associating with a gay person. *Journal of Social Psychology, 131,* 45–56.

Signorella, M. L., Bigler, R. S., & Liben, L. S. (1993). Developmental differences in children's gender schemata about others: A meta-analytic review. *Developmental Review, 13,* 106–126.

Simon, W., & Gagnon, J. H. (1987). A sexual scripts approach. In J. H. Geer & W. T. O'Donoghue (Eds.), *Theories of human sexuality* (pp. 363–383). London: Plenum Press.

Slade, A. (1987). Quality of attachment and early symbolic play. *Developmental Psychology, 23,* 78–85.

Smith, D. (1990). *Stepmothering.* London: Harvester Wheatsheaf.

Smith, P. B., & Pederson, D. (1988). Maternal sensitivity and patterns of infant–mother attachment. *Child Development, 59,* 1097–1101.

Smith, P. K. (1991). The silent nightmare: Bullying and victimisation in school peer groups. *The Psychologist: Bulletin of the British Psychological Society, 4,* 243–248.

Socarides, C. W. (1978). *Homosexuality.* New York: Aronson.

Spielberger, C. (1983). *The handbook of the State–Trait Anxiety Inventory.* Palo Alto, CA: Consulting Psychologists Press.

Sroufe, L. A., Fox, N. E., & Pancake, V. R. (1983). Attachment and dependency in developmental perspective. *Child Development, 54,* 1615–1627.

Stagnor, C., & Ruble, D. N. (1987). Development of gender role knowledge and gender constancy. In L. S. Liben & M. L. Signorella (Eds.), *New directions for child development: No. 38. Children's gender schemata* (pp. 5–22). San Francisco: Jossey-Bass.

Steckel, A. (1987). Psychological development of children of lesbian mothers. In F. W. Bozett (Ed.), *Gay and lesbian parents* (pp. 75–85). New York: Praeger.

Steinberg, L., Lamborn, S. D., Darling, N., Mounts, N. S., & Dornbusch, S. M. (1994). Over-time changes in adjustment and competence among adolescents from authoritative, authoritarian, indulgent and neglectful families. *Child Development, 65,* 754–770.

Stern, M., & Karraker, K. H. (1989). Sex stereotyping of infants: A review of gender labeling studies. *Sex Roles, 20,* 501–522.

Stevenson, M. R., & Black, K. N. (1988). Paternal absence and sex role development: A meta-analysis. *Child Development, 59,* 793–814.

Suess, G. J., Grossmann, K. E., & Sroufe, L. A. (1992). Effects of infant attachment to mother and father on quality of adaptation in preschool: From dyadic to individual organization of self. *International Journal of Behavioral Development, 15,* 43–65.

Svanum, S., Bringle, R. G., & McLaughlin, J. E. (1982). Father absence and cognitive performance in a large sample of six-to-eleven-year-old children. *Child Development, 53,* 136–143.

Tasker, F. L. (1992). Anti-marriage attitudes and motivations to marry amongst adolescents with divorced parents. *Journal of Divorce and Remarriage, 18,* 105–119.

Tasker, F., & Golombok, S. (1991). Children raised by lesbian mothers: The empirical evidence. *Family Law, 21,* 184–187.

Tasker, F., & Golombok, S. (1995). Adults raised as children in lesbian families. *American Journal of Orthopsychiatry, 65,* 203–215.

Tasker, F. L., & Richards, M. P. M. (1994). Adolescents' attitudes toward marriage and marital prospects after parental divorce: A review. *Journal of Adolescent Research, 9,* 340–362.

Tiefer, L. (1987). Social constructionism and the study of human sexuality. In P. Shaver & C. Hendrick (Eds.), *Review of personality and social psychology: Vol. 7. Sex and gender* (pp. 70–94). London: Sage.

Visher, E., & Visher, J. S. (1979). *Stepfamilies: A guide to working with stepparents and stepchildren.* New York: Brunner/Mazel.

Vuchinich, S., Hetherington, E. M., Vuchinich, R., & Clingempeel. W. G. (1991). Parent–child interaction and gender differences in early adolescents' adaptation to stepfamilies. *Developmental Psychology, 27,* 618–626.

Wallerstein, J. S., & Blakeslee, S. (1989). *Second chances: Men, women and children a decade after divorce.* London: Bantam Press.

Wallerstein, J. S., & Corbin, S. B. (1989). Daughters of divorce: Report from a ten-year follow-up. *American Journal of Orthopsychiatry, 59,* 593–604.

Wallerstein, J. S., Corbin, S. B., & Lewis, J. M. (1988). Children of divorce: A 10-Year study. In E. M. Hetherington & J. D. Arasteh (Eds.), *The impact of divorce, single parenting and stepparenting on children* (pp. 197–214). Hillsdale, NJ: Erlbaum.

Wallerstein, J. S., & Kelly, J. B. (1980). *Surviving the breakup: How children and parents cope with divorce.* New York: Basic Books.

Weiss, R. S. (1979). Growing up a little faster: The experience of growing up in a single-parent household. *Journal of Social Issues, 35,* 97–111.

Weitzman, L. J. (1985). *The divorce revolution: The unexpected social and economic consequences for women and children in America.* London: Macmillan.

Wellings, K., & Bradshaw, S. (1994). First intercourse between men and women. In A. M. Johnson, J. Wadsworth, K. Wellings, & J. Field (Eds.), *Sexual attitudes and lifestyles* (pp. 68–109). Oxford, UK: Blackwell Scientific.

Wellings, K., Wadsworth, J., & Johnson, A. (1994). Sexual diversity and homosexual behaviour. In A. M. Johnson, J. Wadsworth, K.

Wellings, & J. Field (Eds.), *Sexual attitudes and lifestyles* (pp. 183–224). Oxford, UK: Blackwell Scientific.

Whitam, F. (1977). Childhood indicators of male homosexuality. *Archives of Sexual Behavior, 6,* 89–96.

Whitney, I., & Smith, P. K. (1993). A survey of the nature and extent of bullying in junior/middle and secondary schools. *Educational Research, 35,* 3–25.

Williams, K., Goodman, M., & Green, R. (1985). Parent–child factors in childhood socialization in girls. *Journal of the American Academy of Child Psychiatry, 26,* 720–731.

Youngblade, L. M., & Belsky, J. (1992). Parent–child antecedents of 5-year-olds' close friendships: A longitudinal analysis. *Developmental Psychology, 28,* 700–713.

Zaslow, M. J. (1988). Sex differences in children's response to divorce: 1. Research methodology and postdivorce family forms. *American Journal of Orthopsychiatry, 58,* 355–378.

Zaslow, M. J. (1989). Sex differences in children's response to divorce: 2. Samples, variables, ages, and sources. *American Journal of Orthopsychiatry, 59,* 118–141.

Zill, N. (1988). Behavior, achievement, and health problems among children in stepfamilies. In E. M. Hetherington & J. D. Arasteh (Eds.), *The impact of divorce, single parenting and stepparenting on children* (pp. 324–368). Hillsdale, NJ: Erlbaum.

Zuger, B. (1984). Early effeminate behavior in boys: Outcome and significance for homosexuality. *Journal of Nervous and Mental Disease, 172,* 90–97.

Index